Make time for

YOGA

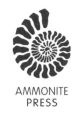

AMMONITE
PRESS

READY TO TRY SOME YOGA?

Lizards, locusts, dogs, bears – yoga can seem baffling, even a little intimidating, at times. But fear not. Our selection of poses, breathing exercises and sequences are designed to help you understand and get started with this ancient practice

Learning a new skill takes time, patience and practice. Yoga is no different. What marks it out, perhaps, is that its physical poses, or *asana*, represent only a fraction of a philosophy that involves life-long learning (page 6).

A low-impact discipline, yoga enhances physical fitness and flexibility, builds strength and resilience, develops awareness of the breath, aids relaxation and nurtures a positive, calm mindset.

This book describes 50 poses, breathing exercises and sequences, which are divided into six sections, Standing, Seated, Supine or Prone, Breathing Exercises, Relaxation, and Flow and Movement.

It's vital to understand how to practise safely (page 12) and warm up (page 18) before moving on to more advanced poses.

Remember, we're all different. Some yogi can twist their core but struggle to touch their toes, others can balance on one leg but find backbends challenging.

Go at your pace. This is your time, your practice, your progress. Thank yourself for caring for your body and mind, and remember, too, to thank the ancient yogis of India and Egypt who bequeathed us this life-affirming philosophy.

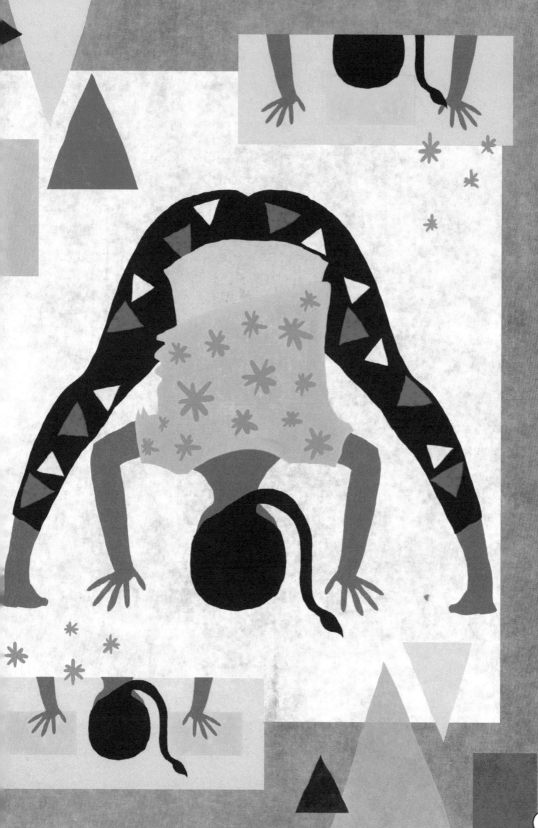

CONTENTS

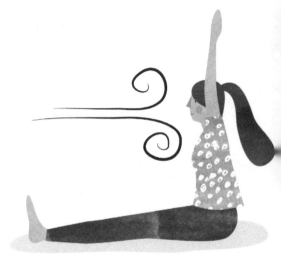

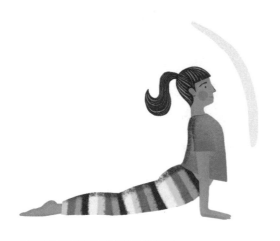

SUPINE/PRONE POSES

BREATHING EXERCISES

RELAXATION

FLOW AND MOVEMENT

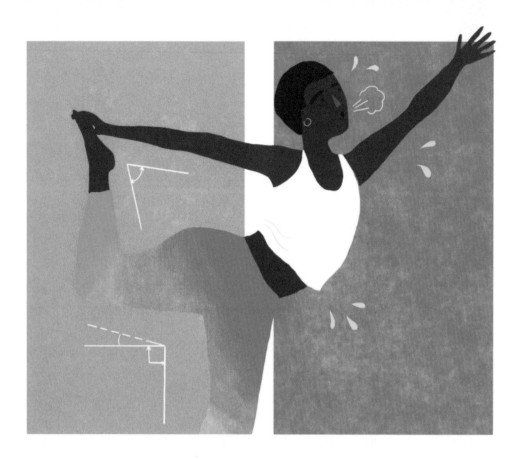

PATH TO ENLIGHTENMENT

The ancient system of yoga goes much deeper than its poses and breathing techniques. Here, we explore some of the lesser-known aspects of the practice

Downward-facing dog, Child's pose, Sun salutation. People the world over enjoy practising these and many other yoga poses and flow sequences. Even non-yogis are familiar with the terminology, such is their popularity.

Not everyone, however, is aware that yoga is far more than a set of stretches, poses and breathing techniques. This ancient practice is a way of living, one with deep spiritual meaning that nurtures mind, body and soul.

The language used to describe its practice and poses, Sanskrit, is found in texts called the *Vedas*, the oldest scriptures in Hinduism. And the Sanskrit noun, *yoga*, means 'yoke', to 'join together' or 'union'. This describes the essence and intention of yoga practice, which is to attain a state of oneness with the divine – where the practitioner's consciousness unites with that of the universe.

The system that's widely practised today is thought to have originated in India about 5,000 years ago. But there's evidence that suggests yoga also has roots in Africa, particularly ancient Egypt.

Here, we explore the wider and deeper meaning of yoga, and the role played by its physical poses.

LIMBS OF YOGA

The practice of yoga comprises eight limbs, which comes from the Sanskrit term *ashtanga*.

This is what each limb involves:

1 Yama

A series of ethical-living rules relating to discipline, which apply to how you behave towards other beings:

* **Ahimsa** – non-violence, freedom from harming. Minimising the amount of harm you are causing to yourself as well as to others in your thoughts, words and actions.
* **Satya** – truthfulness. Before you speak, ask yourself is it true? Is it kind? Is it necessary?
* **Asteya** – non-stealing, freedom from stealing. Not taking that which you have not earned.
* **Brahmacharya** – moderation, avoiding overindulging in pleasures.
* **Aparigraha** – non-hoarding or freedom from grasping. Letting go of unnecessary material attachments.

2 Niyama

These are also a series of ethical-living rules, but this time involving how you conduct yourself on a personal level:

* **Saucha** – cleanliness and purity in relation to your body, mind, environment and company.
* **Santosha** – contentment. Believing you are enough and counting your blessings. Practising gratitude.
* **Tapas** – self-discipline. Transformation through discipline, breaking habitual thought and behaviour.
* **Svadhyaya** – self-study. Being aware of your actions and open to developing wisdom through learning.
* **Isvara pranidhana** – surrender. Giving your energy to something higher than yourself. Letting go of doubt and giving trust to faith.

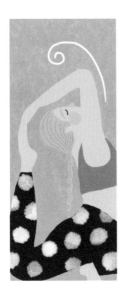
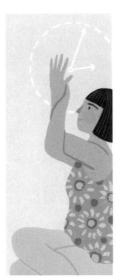
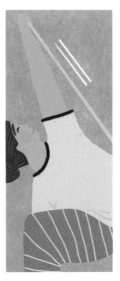
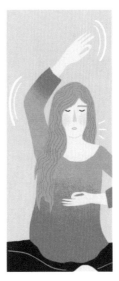

3 Asana

Now we get to the physical practice that most people associate with yoga. *Asana* means 'posture' or 'seat' in Sanskrit and each one helps improve flexibility, strength and balance. They are designed to stimulate the nerves and enhance the function of internal organs and the flow of energy within the body.

Practice of yoga's myriad poses goes hand in hand with breathing (Limb 4, below). Generally, you breathe in when stretching and opening the body, and breathe out when contracting or closing it.

The different poses work with different energy systems within the body. Many are named and constructed from yogic observations of animals, nature and the solar system. Physical practice shouldn't be painful, but rather a gentle exploration that supports the flow of energy within.

4 Pranayama

This is the practice of breath regulation. In Sanskrit, *prana* means 'life-force energy' and *yama* means 'control'. *Pranayama* techniques are designed to improve oxygen flow to the body and the *prana*.

Different breathing techniques have a powerful effect, both physically and mentally. For instance, have you noticed a difference in the way you breathe when you're angry or stressed, compared with when you are calm and happy? In the former state, the breath tends to be shallow and quick. In the latter, it tends to be deeper and slower.

Taking the time to consciously become aware of your breath and its flow within lets you see the way it affects your being and how it can support you in managing both your physical and mental wellbeing.

5 Pratyahara

This is the withdrawal from the senses, or not allowing the senses to determine your actions. For example, dialling down the mind's chatter when it gets distracted by bright lights and sounds, and taking some time to focus inwards in a quiet, tranquil space. This detachment helps to calm and focus the mind.

6 Dharana

In Sanskrit, *dharana* means 'collection' or 'concentration' of the mind. Practice of *dharana* involves bringing your attention to a fixed point, object, mantra or task and being completely focused on what's happening in the present moment.

7 Dhyana

This refers to deeper contemplation and meditation. Where *dharana* teaches one-pointed focus, *dhyana* brings awareness without that single point of attachment. It's more an abstract awareness of everything just as it is.

8 Samadhi

The final stage on the eightfold path of yoga, often referred to as the luminous mind. It's described as a state of bliss and oneness with the divine or the universe.

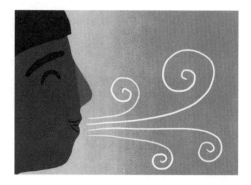

TYPES OF YOGA

Here are four important dimensions in yoga:

Karma – teaches the path of selfless service, detachment from personal gain or recognition. All actions are carried out with a sense of oneness, acting for the greater good of all.

Bhakti – focuses on expressing devotion to a chosen form of the divine, with chanting, singing and ritual devotion.

Raja – calms the mind through meditation and the eightfold path of yoga. *Ashtanga* is a practice of Raja yoga.

Jnana – pursues knowledge through the study of sacred texts and self-enquiry to produce insight and self-realisation.

From this brief overview, it's clear that yoga is a vast and comprehensive system, with many benefits for a practitioner to experience. Have fun exploring it and try not to get too focused on achieving complex or advanced poses, as these physical aspects make up only one of eight limbs.

Remember that the final limb – *samadhi* – is achieved through giving equal attention to each of the other seven.

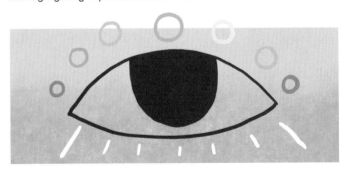

KNOW YOUR KIT

One of the many great things about yoga is that it doesn't need lots of expensive equipment. In fact, for many poses, all that's required is some comfy clothing and a level, non-slip patch of ground or wall-to-wall carpet. Some poses might be made more physically comfortable with the addition of a few basic and inexpensive props. Here, we highlight the essentials.

Mat

Think of yoga and the image of a yogi practising Warrior I pose (page 38) on a long rectangular mat often comes to mind. Traditionally, many yogis practised in their bare feet on hard, flat floors, but a slip-resistant mat is recommended, as it provides cushioning and safety. Many are made of PVC, foam or a mixture of materials. There are also more eco-aware options made of jute or cotton. Always position them on a flat, even surface that is stable and on which they won't slip.

Block

Rectangular in shape and available in materials including plastic, PVC, foam, wood or more environmentally friendly cork, blocks are often used to help extend your reach (in Standing forward bend, for example, page 24), find a comfortable resting point for the forehead (say, in Child's pose, page 108) or raise the bottom in seated poses, such as Butterfly (page 46). There are different sizes, so you may wish to ask a yogi friend if you could try their block before making a purchase.

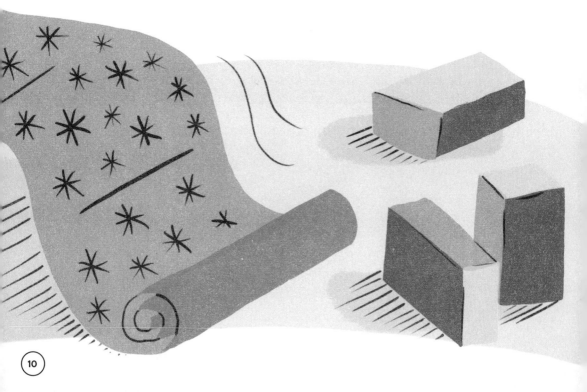

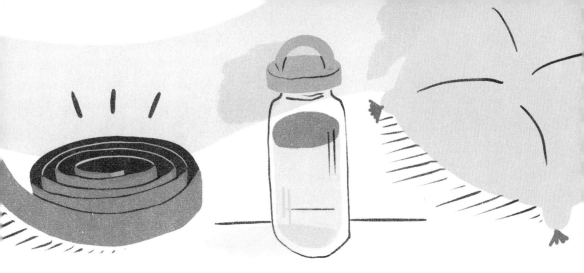

Strap

Generally made of hemp or cotton, they help ease the strain on muscles and are useful for extending reach in poses such as Sitting forward bend (page 52).

Cushion

Any shape, any size (it could even be a pillow or a bolster), but choose one that feels comfortable and enables you to remain comfortably in relaxing poses such as Reclining butterfly (page 68) or Corpse pose (page 114).

Towel

A good-sized cotton sweat towel, or a hand towel if practising at home, is useful to wipe away any moisture that might remain on your mat between poses. This will keep you comfortable and your practice safe.

Water

It's important to stay hydrated during any physical exercise, and that includes yoga. Make sure to top up your water levels before you begin to feel thirsty, particularly during warm weather or if practising in a room where it's difficult to regulate the temperature.

Sweat top or small blanket

Periods of relaxation (for example, Legs up the wall, page 112) and breathing practice (say, Box breathing, page 104) are great for body, mind and spirit. To get the most out of them, it's best that your practice space isn't too hot or cold. A sweat top is ideal if the room's a little chillier than you'd like.

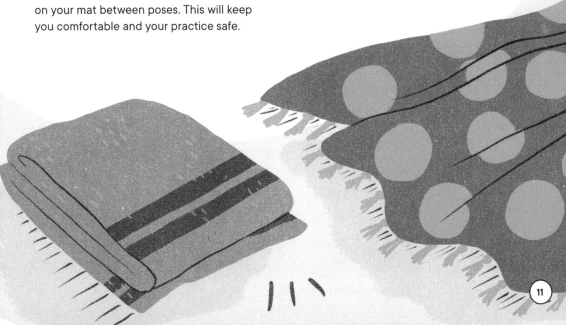

HOW TO PRACTISE SAFELY

The physical poses of yoga might only be a small part of this age-old philosophy, but it's vital to practise them safely and approach them with a gentle and attentive mindset. It's the process that matters, not the end goal. Everyone's body is built differently and people have varying levels of flexibility, so focus on what feels right for you. Here are a few pointers for a safe, nurturing practice. As a general guide, most poses begin on the right side of the body.

* Practise on an empty stomach, so maybe before breakfast or late evening, but at least two hours after eating a light lunch or dinner.

* Try to stick to a routine – maybe half an hour once a week on a Saturday morning, or 15-20 minutes three times a week on a Tuesday, Thursday and Sunday evening. See what works for you. But don't be down on yourself if you miss a day. Sometimes, it's just not possible to fit everything in. You might also skip practice for a while, and that's OK, too. You can start practising again when it feels right for you.

* Create a space that is calm and quiet, somewhere you won't be distracted.

* Aim to be in a room that's neither too hot nor too cold. If you practise outdoors during warmer weather, make sure you're not in direct sunlight.

* Breathe steadily through the poses, and try to keep the face relaxed.

* Never push your body beyond what feels comfortable. Don't stretch too far and don't twist too far. Yoga shouldn't involve pain.

* Pay special attention to your back. Everyone's back is different and has its own twinges and weaker points, so don't force yours into a position where it doesn't feel right or it hurts.

* Be careful with balance poses. It's wise to practise them by a wall for support.

* Use whatever props and kit you need to keep your body safe.

* Build your practice slowly and surely, starting with beginner poses and moving on only when it feels comfortable and safe to do so.

* Include counter-poses in your practice, which means to take the body in the opposite direction. If, for example, you spend time in a backbend, you might follow it up with a gentle forward bend.

* Stop if you feel tired. Also stop immediately if you feel dizzy, in pain, nauseous or out of breath. The aim of yoga isn't to exhaust or hurt yourself, it's to enjoy your practice.

* For female practitioners, the deep breathing during yoga encourages the circulation of oxygen to the muscles, which can help soothe menstrual cramps. When you have your period, it's good to keep the body aligned to the direction of the energetic flow of menstruation. For this reason, avoid poses that put your uterus in the air or upside-down during menstruation.

* It's not advisable to begin yoga during pregnancy. If you're already attending a class, let your teacher know. For home practice, take care not to perform poses that constrict the abdomen, and never become fatigued or breathless. Of the poses featured in this book, do not attempt any that put pressure on the abdomen or involve deep twists, lying flat on your back or belly, backbends, crunches and inversions. It's always advisable to talk to your GP.

* Do not attempt any poses if you have any medical conditions or injuries that might be aggravated. If in any doubt, consult with a health professional first.

* Younger practitioners should always be supervised.

* If you can, try to attend a class with a qualified and nurturing yoga teacher, who will guide your physical practice and give you a greater understanding of the wider spiritual benefits of yoga.

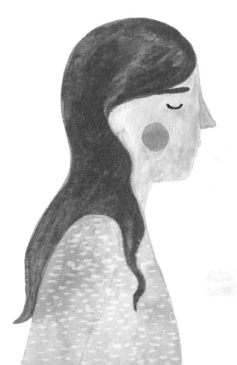

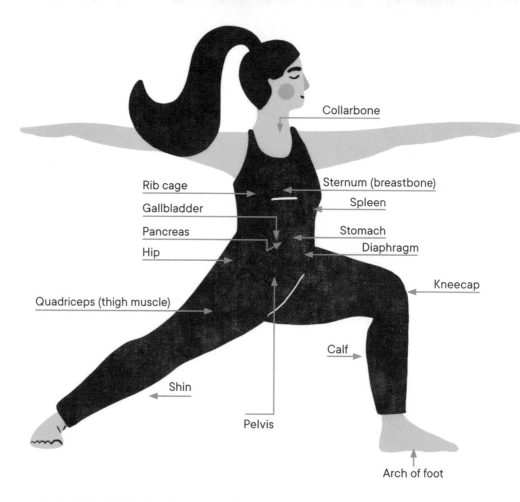

Collarbone

Rib cage

Sternum (breastbone)

Gallbladder

Spleen

Pancreas

Stomach

Hip

Diaphragm

Kneecap

Quadriceps (thigh muscle)

Calf

Shin

Pelvis

Arch of foot

ALIGNMENT OF THE SELF

Knowing how to hold your body safely and assuredly will enable you to get the most out of your practice

Just as the philosophy of yoga aims for union and alignment with universal consciousness or the cosmos (page 6), the physical practice of poses encourages awareness and appreciation of every part of the body – limbs, internal organs, joints, muscles, cells, skin, breath – and how they combine and align in movement.

An understanding of the body's anatomy is important (see images, above), but the key to enjoying a fulfilling and beneficial practice lies in becoming conscious of the body's alignment in each pose. This improves the effectiveness of each one and reduces the risk of injury.

A general principle is that joints are stacked over each other vertically, with body parts aligned in relation to each other. This brings physical balance by maintaining the natural shape and placement of inner organs, creates internal space to deepen the breath and helps to increase the flow of energy while also calming the mind.

Alignment begins at the base, so ensure you're rooted into the earth by pushing

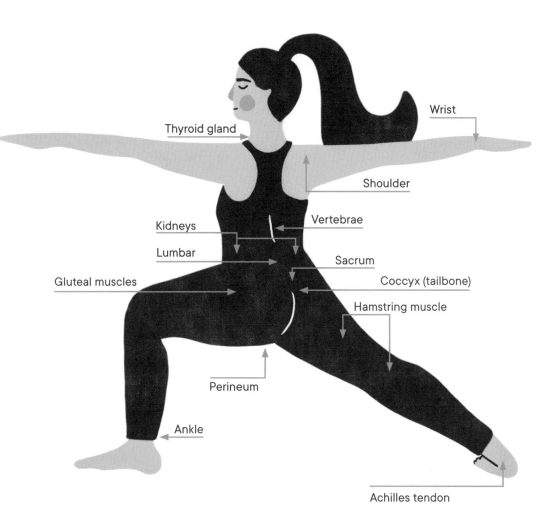

Thyroid gland

Wrist

Shoulder

Kidneys

Vertebrae

Lumbar

Sacrum

Gluteal muscles

Coccyx (tailbone)

Hamstring muscle

Perineum

Ankle

Achilles tendon

down through the feet and aligning them in relation to the hips, shoulders and arms, be that vertically, for example in Mountain pose (page 22), or horizontally in, say, Warrior II (images above and page 40) or Triangle (page 26).

Consciously engage the muscle groups described for each pose, bring awareness to your core, lower the shoulders, keep the head in line with the neck and pay attention to your breath.

Another tip is to resist overworking areas that feel naturally flexible and to try to keep your back straight by bending at the hip, for example, in Standing forward bend (page 24).

Full alignment also requires balance, so poses are always practised on both sides of the body. So, if you start on the right leg in Sun salutation (page 116), you need to repeat the sequence on the left.

With practice, it's possible to build on this awareness, bring flow into the poses, regulate the breath and find inner calm. It might also become easier to remember to soften the face and smile, too.

EVERYTHING BEGINS AND ENDS WITH THE BREATH

When we are born, we naturally breathe deeply. If you observe a baby sleeping, you can see their breaths are deep and go all the way down to their belly – watch and see how their tummy clearly rises and falls with the breath. As we grow up, this breathing pattern changes – some estimates suggest adults use only 20% of their lung capacity. Luckily, all is not lost. It's possible to re-establish that deep breathing by bringing conscious awareness to the breath, which will prove beneficial in everyday life as well as yoga practice.

Here's how to bring conscious awareness to the breath:

1. Lie on your back on the floor. Begin with the arms in a relaxed position beside the body, palms facing upwards, with your legs falling loosely away from each other.

2. Gently close your eyes and take a few moments to get comfortable and settle your mind and body. Gently and steadily breathe in and out through your nostrils.

3. Now start to bring greater awareness to your breath, as you prepare to practise conscious breathwork, using a 1:2 ratio. This means making the out-breath twice as long as the in-breath.

4. Take a deep breath in through your nose for a count of three, breathe it in all the way down to your stomach – allow your stomach to expand with the breath. It's sometimes helpful to place one hand on your heart and the other on your stomach, so that you can feel the rise and fall as you breathe in and out.

5. Hold the breath for as long as comfortable, say a count of two, then slowly breathe out for a count of six. Repeat this breathing pattern for three to five minutes and observe how your body and mind feel afterwards. You may find they're more peaceful and relaxed.

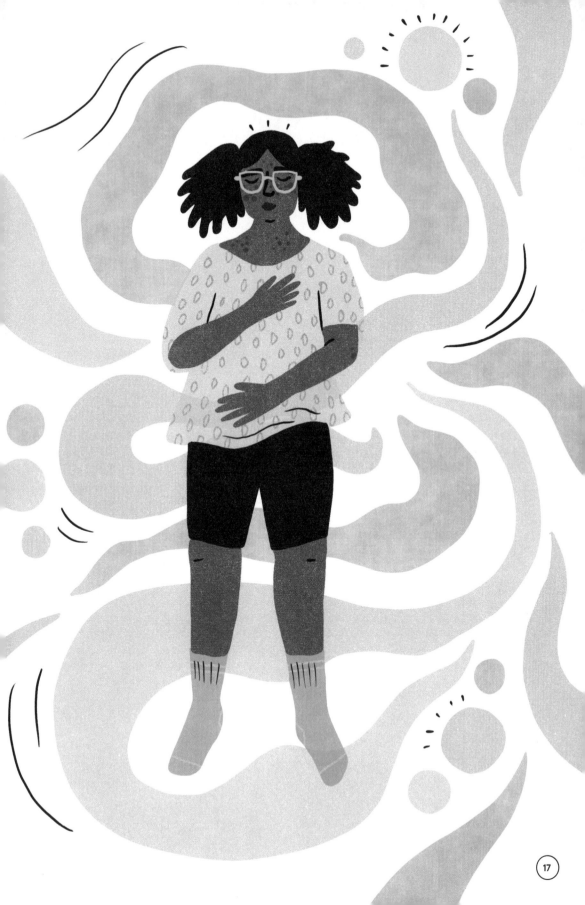

THE ESSENTIAL WARM-UP

Before engaging in any physical exercise, it's sensible to warm up the body. This applies as much to practising yoga poses as it does going out for a run. A gentle warm-up will increase blood and fluid circulation. It will also loosen muscles and joints, making them more flexible and less susceptible to injury.

Harnessing the breath during your warm-up will boost the supply of oxygen and blood flow to the muscles, which will also support more efficient movement. There are many different warm-up exercises and routines. This sequence can be used ahead of easing yourself into gentle poses.

Here's how to practise your warm-up:

1. Begin by lying flat on the ground in Corpse pose (page 114), arms loosely by the side of the body with palms up, feet softly tipping outwards. Take a few moments to breathe here and connect with your breath, mind and body. Breathe in deeply through your nose, take the breath down to your stomach, and then breathe out slowly through your nose. On an in-breath, raise your arms alongside your head extending backwards, while also stretching your toes as far forwards as you can – imagine you're being pulled in opposite directions through your arms and legs.

2. On an in-breath, bend your right knee and slowly bring it towards your chest. Wrap your arms around it and give it a hug, breathing in. Then draw your head towards your knee and, if you are able to reach, give it a kiss.

3. On an out-breath, gently lower your head back to the ground. Take hold of your right toe or ankle with your right hand and extend your leg straight towards the sky, feeling the stretch along the back of your leg (it's OK to have a bend in the knee if this is more comfortable. You can also wrap your hands around the back of the right thigh). Hold for a moment before releasing and slowly lowering the extended leg to the ground. Repeat the sequence with the left leg.

4. Now bend both knees, bring them to the chest, hug them and gently rock back and forth on your back to come up carefully to a cross-legged seated position.

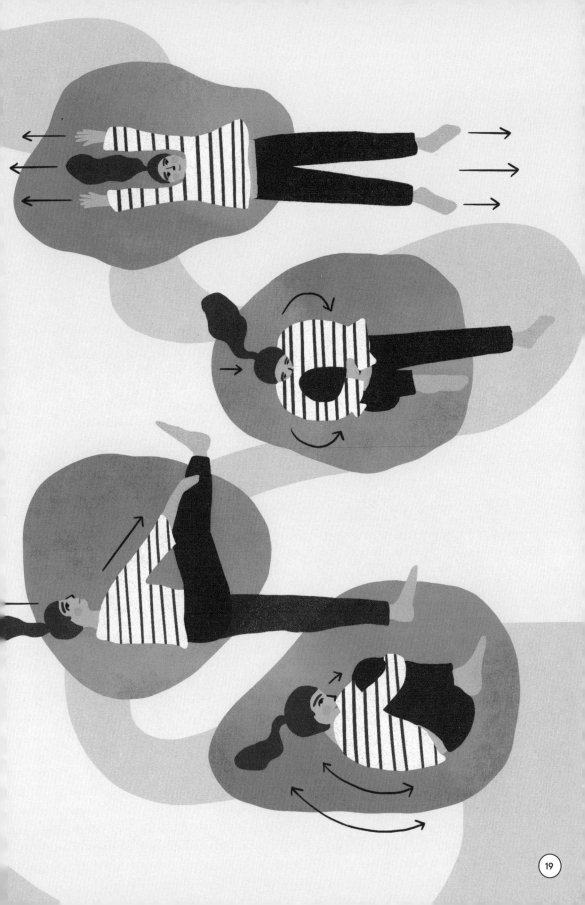

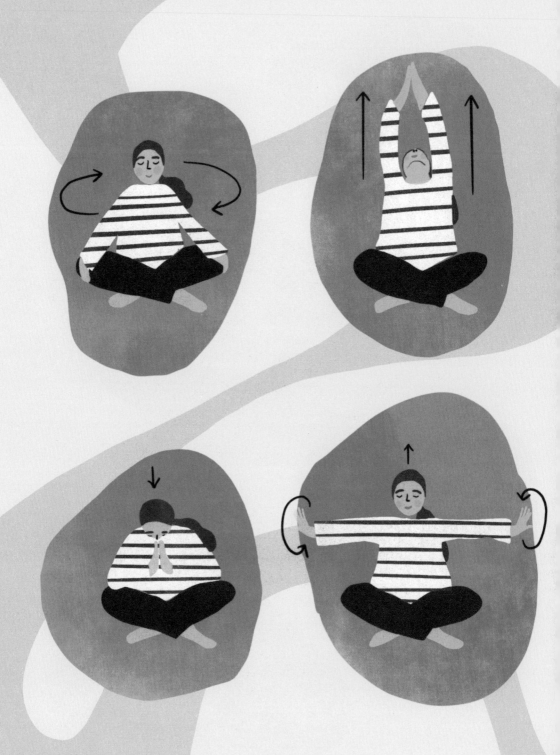

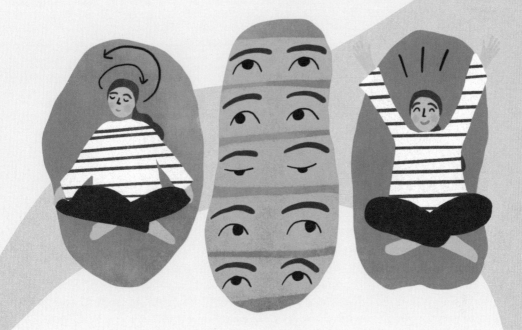

5. Place your hands on your knees. On an in-breath, extend your upper torso forwards from the hips and begin to draw a circle in a clockwise direction. Breathe out as the circle extends backwards. Do this five times. Then repeat the process in the opposite direction, so anticlockwise, remembering to move from the hips. At the end, come to your centre, sitting upright and tall.

6. Bring hands together at heart centre in Prayer pose (elbows active and pushed out from the chest, palms softly pressing together, fingers pointed up). On an in-breath, raise your hands skywards, keeping the palms together. Direct the gaze upwards to follow the hands. Take a moment before breathing out as you lower your hands back to your chest. Now bring the chest forwards, and lower your head and chin towards it. Repeat five times.

7. Release your hands. Extend them sideways from the shoulders and gently rotate your wrists clockwise three times, then anticlockwise three times. Follow

this with three gentle wrist flexes up and down. Do this by first holding out the right arm level with the shoulder, then point the right hand down towards the floor (palm towards you) and hold for a breath. Now turn the hand upwards, fingers pointing to the ceiling (palm facing away). You may choose to use your opposite hand to keep the flexed wrist gently in position. Repeat the sequence on the left wrist.

8. Bring your hands to rest on your knees and slowly make three small circles with your head, first clockwise and then anticlockwise.

9. Looking directly ahead, gently warm up your eyeballs. Without moving your head, direct your eyes to gaze first skywards, then right, then to the floor, then left before coming back to the sky. Repeat in the opposite direction.

10. Your body will feel gently warmed and your muscles and joints will have more flexibility as you begin your practice. Your mind, too, will be in a more restful place.

MOUNTAIN

Tadasana

Although it might look like you're just standing still, there's a lot going on in this pose, which is the foundation for all standing poses and sequences. It should feel easy and comfortable for you to hold for some time, while providing a strong and stable base. This is great for becoming centred and aware of the body's position – keep in mind how the joints are stacked over each other vertically (page 14). Mountain pose is particularly effective for ensuring proper alignment of the hands in relation to the rest of the body.

Here's how to explore the pose:

1. Stand with feet hip-width apart and parallel, toes pointing forwards, knees facing forwards and in line with the ankles.

2. Visualise grounding down through the feet, but avoid collapsing the body.

3. Keeping the knees soft, visualise a gentle opening across the backs of them, creating a sense of lengthening up and down the legs.

4. Allow the arms to fall naturally and lightly by the sides of the body. The biceps and thumbs face forwards while the palms face the thighs.

5. Visualise a thread passing through the body, from the soles of the feet and up through the crown of the head.

6. Let the thread create lightness in the upper body – a gentle elongation from the waist up.

7. While remaining alert and aware of the position of the body, relax into a rhythm of calm breathing. Remain here for at least one minute.

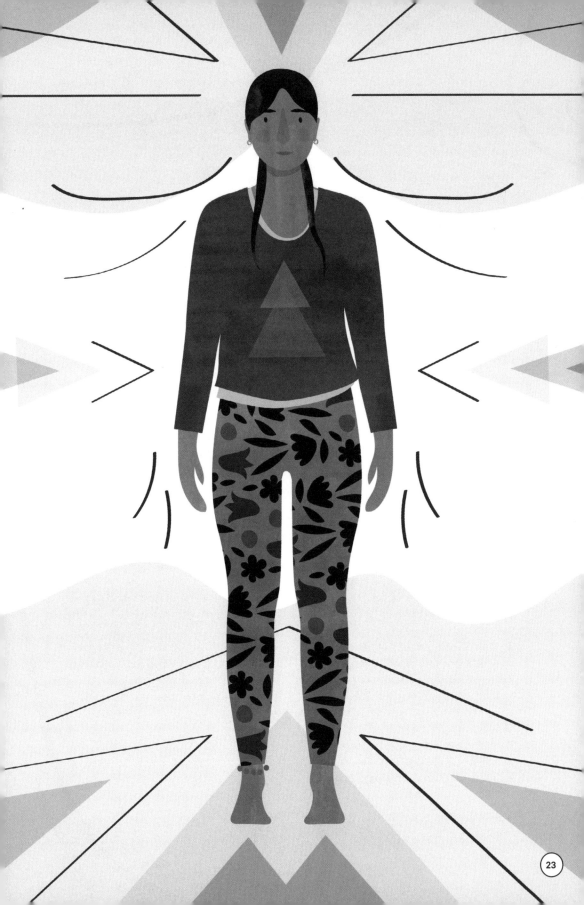

STANDING FORWARD BEND

Uttanasana

A yoga pose that helps to release internal tension, Standing forward bend is considered to be stress-relieving and relaxing. It lengthens the hamstrings and stretches the back, releasing compression and tension in the vertebrae (the small bones in the back), calming the mind and rejuvenating the body.

Here's how to explore the pose:

1. Stand tall and upright, feet hip-width apart, with feet, knees and hips aligned and facing forwards. Take a few deep breaths, raising the crown of your head skywards, allowing your shoulders to relax back and down, and the chest to open forwards.

2. On an in-breath raise your arms, so they're pointing straight up, palms facing each other. Take a few deep breaths, gently lengthening your spine upwards with each in-breath.

3. On an out-breath, fold forwards from your hips (not your waist), and gently release your upper body towards the floor, keeping your back straight. The knees should be soft and not locked. Bring your palms to rest on the floor beside your feet. (You may need to bend your knees to maintain a straight back. You could also rest your hands on a yoga block.)

4. Take a few deep breaths in this position. Explore how your body feels as you release and expand your vertebrae downwards, head and neck gently releasing towards the earth.

5. To come out of this position, on an in-breath, push down through your legs and, from the hips, slowly raise your torso – vertebrae by vertebrae – with your head coming up last to a standing-tall position and arms coming up and round to gently rest alongside your torso.

6. Take a few deep breaths and observe the effect this pose has on your being, noting any new-found spaciousness within, a release of tension or peace of mind.

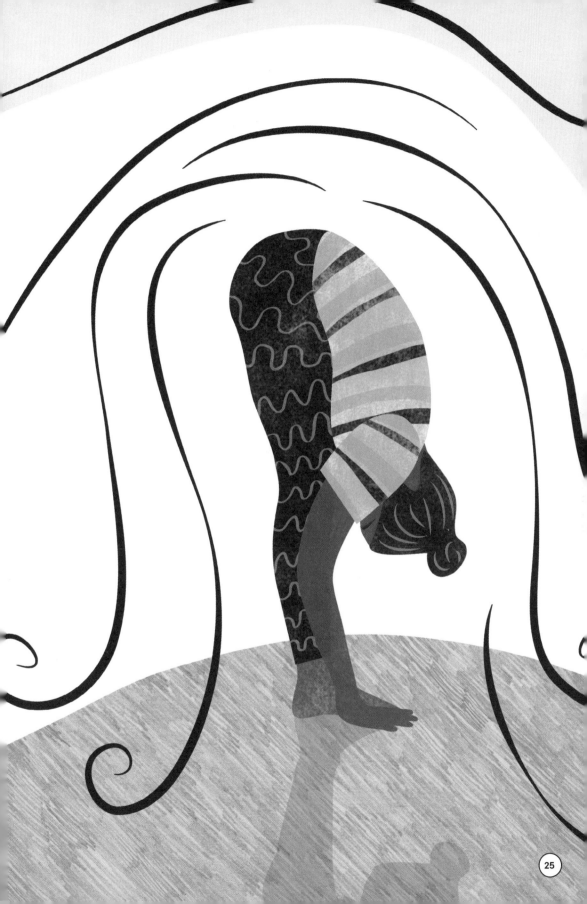

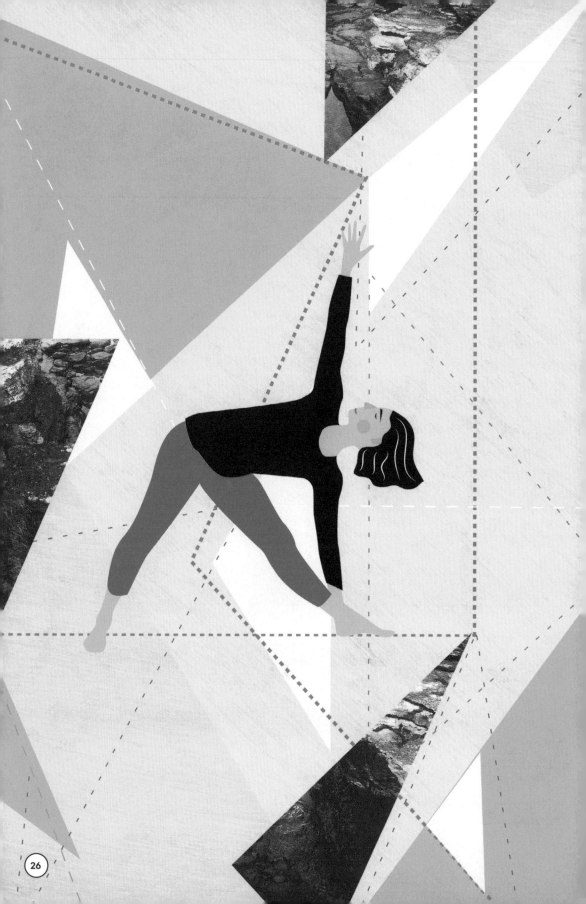

TRIANGLE

Trikonasana

Triangles are considered the strongest geometric shape as they absorb any additional force evenly throughout their three sides. In yoga, Triangle also has a strong geometric quality. Great for core strength, it also builds flexibility and stamina in the legs, hips and torso.

Here's how to explore the pose:

1. Stand tall, feet hip-width apart. Take a few deep breaths.

2. On an out-breath, step your feet out wide to the sides. Raise both arms to shoulder level, parallel to the floor with the palms facing down, and extend outwards through your fingers, as in Warrior II (page 40). Now is a good time to adjust the distance between your feet – the ankle should be directly below the wrist on each of your outstretched arms.

3. Lift your torso, lengthening both sides of your waist, then broaden your chest and lengthen your neck.

4. Turn your left leg out from the hip socket, so that your foot is at 90 degrees to your body. Turn the toes of your right foot in slightly.

5. On an out-breath, extend to the left and gently fold into your left hip socket. Lower your left arm so the hand rests on the floor outside of your left foot. If this feels awkward, try placing your hand on your shin, ankle or a yoga block – wherever is most comfortable for you.

6. Raise your right arm straight up skywards in line with your shoulders, palms open in the frontward direction. Open your chest and shoulders wide. Now, a straight line has been formed between both arms.

7. Lengthen your neck to look either upwards towards your hand or straight ahead, whichever is most comfortable.

8. Take a few deep breaths here, maintaining the length in both sides of your body while trying not to crunch over onto the left.

9. To come out of the pose, on an in-breath, push down through the legs, raise your torso back to standing with arms back to parallel position. Step your feet together and lower the arms to your side.

10. Take a few breaths here. When ready, repeat the sequence, this time leading with your right leg.

WIDE-LEGGED FORWARD BEND

Prasarita padottanasana

Strengthen the legs, hips, lower back, spine, abdominal region and chest with Wide-legged forward bend. The Sanskrit term can be broken down into five elements: *prasarita* means 'spread' or 'expanded', *pada* is 'foot' or 'leg', *utta* is 'intense', *tan* is 'stretch' and *asana* is 'seat', 'place' or 'pose'. As well as providing a powerful stretch, it helps to release tension and calm the mind.

Here's how to explore the pose:

1. Stand tall, with your head and torso lifting upwards and facing forwards, and your hands alongside your body in Mountain pose (page 22). Take a few breaths to ground and centre your being.

2. Raise your arms so they come level with the shoulders. Keep the arms parallel to the floor, palms facing downwards, as in Warrior II (page 40). On an in-breath, step your feet wide apart. A good reference point is to align the ankles below the wrists of your extended arms.

3. Lower the hands and rest them on your hips. Ground yourself by pressing into your big toes and the balls of your feet. On an in-breath, lift your chest, roll your shoulder blades back and down, and open your chest area. At the same time, engage your thigh muscles and your core.

4. On an out-breath, fold forwards from your hips to a position where your torso is parallel to the floor. Take your hands and place them flat on the ground below your shoulders. Your tailbone is lifted and the torso extends forwards, legs straight. You might find it helpful to rest your hands on some yoga blocks (see inset, bottom left). Take a few breaths here.

5. If it feels comfortable to go further into the fold (remember, it's important to maintain a straight back), bend the elbows and walk the hands back to a position parallel to the feet. The crown of the head reaches towards the ground. If possible, rest the crown of the head on the ground or a block (see inset, top right). Bend the knees a little if this feels in any way uncomfortable, and be careful not to push yourself too far. Take a few steady breaths.

6. To come out of the pose, walk the hands forwards to the half-fold position, then return them to the hips. Engaging the leg and stomach muscles – and working from the hips – return the torso to an upright position, step your feet together and release your hands to sit alongside the body.

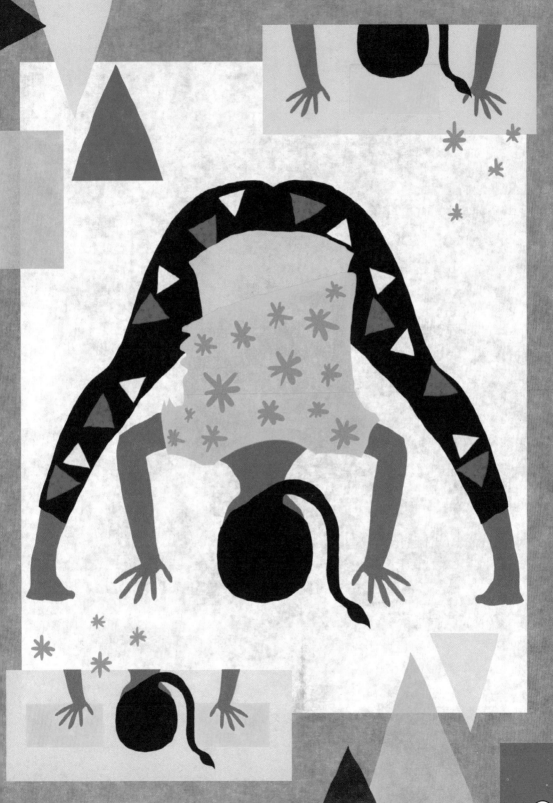

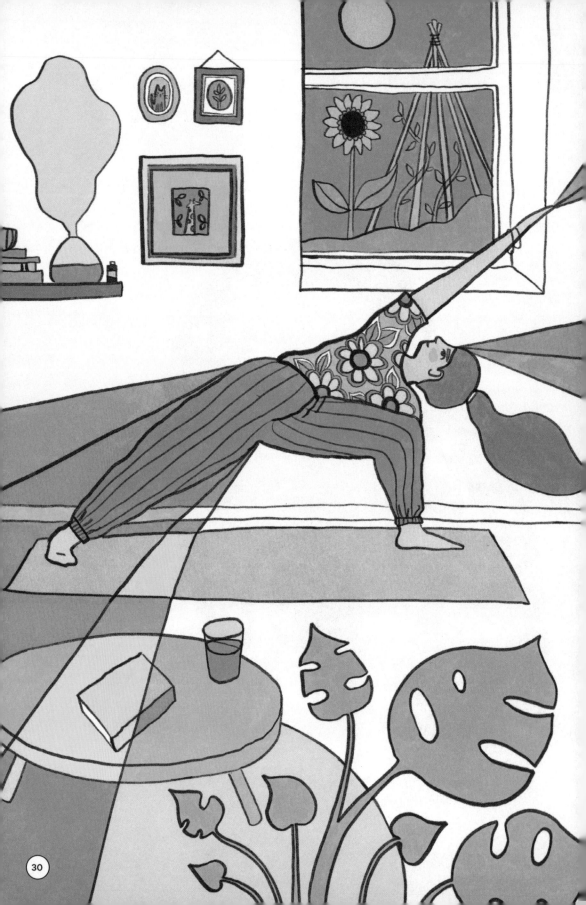

EXTENDED SIDE-ANGLE STRETCH

Utthita parsvakonasana

Embrace the mindset that strength lies in flexibility with Extended side angle stretch, which is also known as Warrior angle pose. This pose provides many benefits, harnessing the strength of Warrior II (page 40) with the freedom of space through the extension of both sides of the body. It boosts energy and improves balance and posture, helping to counteract the effects of sitting still for too long. It also strengthens the legs, hips and hamstrings, stimulates digestion and opens the chest and shoulders.

Here's how to explore the pose:

1. To begin, stand tall, with your shoulders rolled back and down, and your chest wide and open. Take a moment to breathe, connect with your inner strength and set your intention for the pose.

2. On an in-breath, extend your arms out from your shoulders horizontally, palms open and facing downwards. Jump or step your feet apart so that your ankles are roughly below your wrists.

3. Turn your left leg out at 90 degrees, so your toes and knees are pointing in the same direction as your extended fingers. Turn your right foot slightly inwards.

4. On an in-breath, engage the muscles in your legs and core, pressing downwards through both legs. On an out-breath, bend your left knee into a 90-degrees lunge, with your left thigh parallel to the floor. Your right leg remains straight.

5. On another in-breath lift your torso, then, moving from your hips, lean to the side, so your torso is over your left knee. Bring your left hand to rest on the ground outside your left foot. If this is difficult, rest your hand on a block or against your calf. Only bend as far as feels comfortable.

6. Reach your right arm up over your head, palm facing the floor, so that your extended arm forms a straight line running all the way up your right leg to the tips of your fingers. Open your chest and look up at your right palm. Breathe here for a few comfortable breaths.

7. On an out-breath, flow your right arm back towards the right foot, press through both legs and, working from the hips, bring your torso to upright. At the same time, straighten your left leg and bring the arms back to parallel with the floor. Take a few breaths. Repeat on the opposite side.

PEACEFUL WARRIOR

Shanti virabhadrasana

As the name suggests, Peaceful warrior brings calm and tranquillity to the mind while channelling the inner fortitude of a warrior to the body. This powerful side-bend activates the muscles in the legs and opens the heart and chest area, aiding respiratory functions and increasing energy flow. It strengthens the core and releases tension in the shoulders, arms and neck. It is through this combination of flexibility and balance that peace is attained.

Here's how to explore the pose:

1. Stand tall in Mountain pose (page 22) at the centre of your yoga mat. Take a moment to breathe and connect with your inner strength and peace.

2. Come into Warrior II (page 40) by stepping out with your right leg and bending the knee, pointing the toes of your right foot towards the front of the mat, your right knee aligned above your right ankle. Your left leg is straight, toes pointing towards the upper-left corner of your mat.

3. Raise your arms level with the shoulders, as in Warrior II, before stretching your right arm forwards (in the direction of the front of your mat), while at the same time reaching backwards with your left (your torso faces in the direction of your outstretched right arm).

4. Turn the palm of your right hand to face upwards. On an in-breath, raise your right hand skywards, extending through the right of the torso from the hips.

5. On an out-breath, lower your left hand, extending through your left side until the hand comes to rest gently on your left thigh (or lower down the leg if comfortable). At the same time, extend the right side of your body up and over, towards the back of your mat, to create a leftward lean.

6. As you maintain the length on both sides of your body throughout the stretch (the gaze is directed skywards towards your right hand), be aware of the shoulders gently opening backwards and the chest staying open. Keep the extension through your spine and neck.

7. Take a few comfortable breaths. On an in-breath, return to Warrior II, then to Mountain pose. Breathe. Repeat on the opposite side to achieve full body balance.

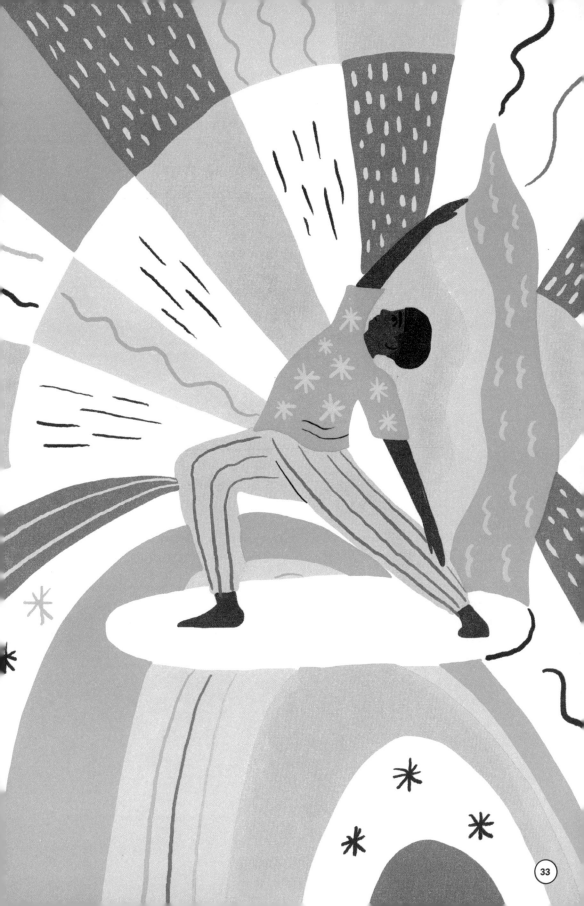

TREE

Vrksasana

Have you ever stopped to observe a tree? It stands tall and strong, rooted in the ground, surviving all seasons. Practising Tree pose helps you to stand equally as tall and strong. A grounding posture, it brings peace and calm to the mind and body while lengthening the spine and strengthening the calves and ankles.

Here's how to explore the pose:

1. Stand with your arms by your side – palms open and facing forwards. Take a moment to breathe deeply, connect with your core and ground your feet with the earth below.

2. On an in-breath, bring your hands into Prayer position at the heart centre (Step 6, page 21). Take a few breaths to enjoy the peace and calm of this position.

3. Shift your weight onto your right foot. Imagine it has strong, deep roots growing into the ground.

4. Bend your left knee and gently place the sole of your left foot against your right leg – you can use your hand to guide the foot. It can be on the inner thigh, along the lower part of the leg or anywhere that feels comfortable, but NEVER against the knee (this can cause injury). Some yogis place the foot with their toes resting on the floor and the sole against the right ankle.

5. On an out-breath, raise your arms – keeping the palms in Prayer position – above your head. Take a few deep breaths here, with chest and shoulders open wide and legs strong and grounded.

6. Slowly lower your arms to return to Prayer pose at the heart centre, then lower your left foot back to standing position.

7. Take a moment to observe how your body feels. Now repeat the exercise on the other side of the body, grounding through your left leg and bringing the right foot to the left thigh.

8. Practising Tree pose on both sides brings balance to your body. Stay grounded and you will soon be as strong, tall and majestic as a mighty oak.

Tips:
* If you feel unsteady, open the arms wide to help maintain balance.
* To maintain focus, keep your eyes open and direct your gaze towards a fixed object directly ahead of you.

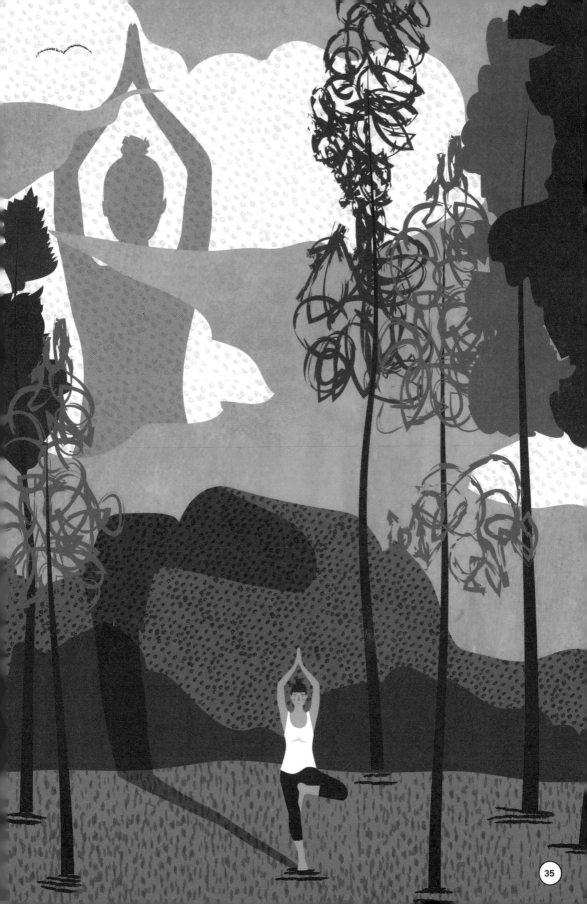

EAGLE

Garudasana

Eagles are admired as symbols of power, freedom and transcendence. They're strong, proud, noble creatures with amazing eyesight – they can spy prey more than 3km away. Eagle pose is a standing balance that develops personal focus, strength and serenity. It stretches the shoulders and upper back, which, in turn, increases breathing capacity and strengthens the thighs, hips, ankles and calves. Anyone with knee injuries is advised to avoid this pose or follow the alternative option as described in our tips (see below).

Here's how to explore the pose:

1. Stand strong in Mountain pose (page 22). Aim to be tall, with your chest out, shoulders down, feet forwards and arms beside the body, palms forwards.

2. On an in-breath, extend your arms straight ahead in front of you at shoulder level. Keep your palms facing upwards.

3. Cross your left arm over your right arm. Bend your arms at the elbow and wrap your forearms around each other, bringing your palms together and pointing the hands up towards the sky. (You can also have the backs of your hands touching if that feels more comfortable.)

4. On an out-breath, slightly bend your knees and shift your body weight onto your left leg.

5. On an in-breath, cross your right thigh and knee over your left, and hook your right foot behind your left calf.

6. Hold this position, breathing in and out slowly and deeply. As you balance, feel yourself calm, focused, strong and proud, just like an eagle.

7. On an out-breath, release your limbs back into Mountain pose.

8. Breathe and reground yourself before repeating the pose, remembering to begin with your opposite arm and leg to balance out the body.

9. If you practise Eagle regularly, you'll be able to observe how your balance, focus, strength and serenity begin to soar.

Tips:
* To assist balance, focus your gaze on a stationary point in front of you.
* Use a wall to brace and support your back while learning to balance.
* It can be difficult to hook the foot of the raised leg behind the calf of the standing one and still maintain balance. An alternative option is to cross the legs but, instead of hooking the raised foot behind the calf of the standing leg, press the big toe of the raised foot against the floor to help with stability.

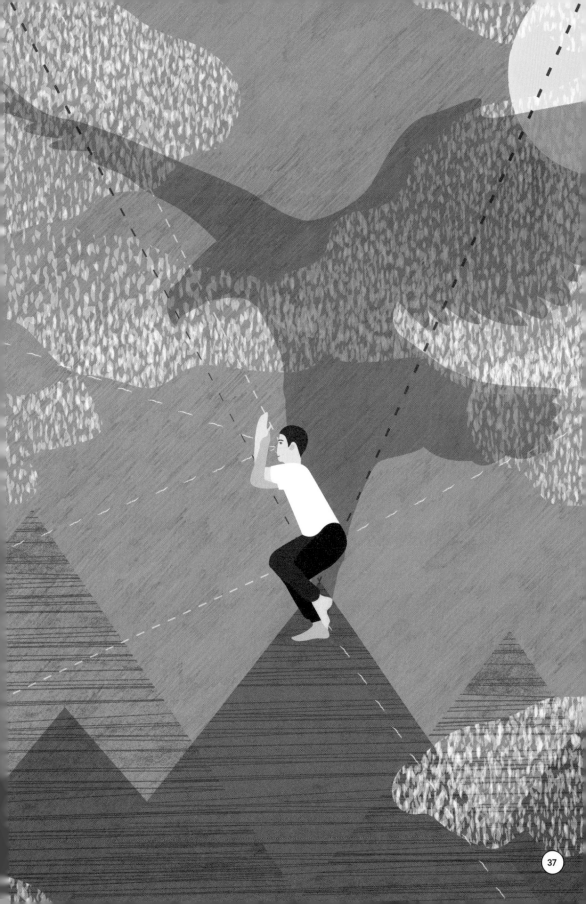

WARRIOR I
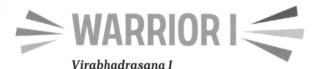

Virabhadrasana I

Warrior supports us in stepping forward in our greatness and following our passions in life. It has several variations. Warrior I, described here, strengthens the legs, opens the hips and chest, and stretches the arms and legs. It also helps to develop strength, confidence, concentration, balance and stability.

Here's how to explore the pose:

1. Stand tall in Mountain pose (page 22) with your feet hip-distance apart and your arms at your side. Take a few deep breaths here and feel the ground supporting you. Take time to connect to your core within.

2. On an out-breath, step your feet wide apart (to a point that's comfortable). Turn your right leg and foot out by 90 degrees. Turn the left foot in slightly, to about 40 degrees. The heels of the feet should be aligned with each other. Swing your hips around to face your right leg, bringing your torso to face in the same direction. On an in-breath, lift your arms up over your head, stretching skywards with your palms facing each other. Take a few breaths.

3. On an out-breath, lower your tailbone (that's the bone at the bottom of your spine) towards the ground and bend your right leg into a deep lunge. Your right knee aligns directly over your right ankle and your right thigh comes parallel to the ground, forming the shape of a right angle.

4. Look up or forwards, lifting your torso upwards, while at the same time pushing downwards through your tailbone and legs. Take a few deep breaths.

5. To come out of the pose, slowly straighten your right leg, turn both feet forwards, lower the arms and step back into Mountain pose. Take a moment to observe how you feel and then repeat the above for the opposite leg.

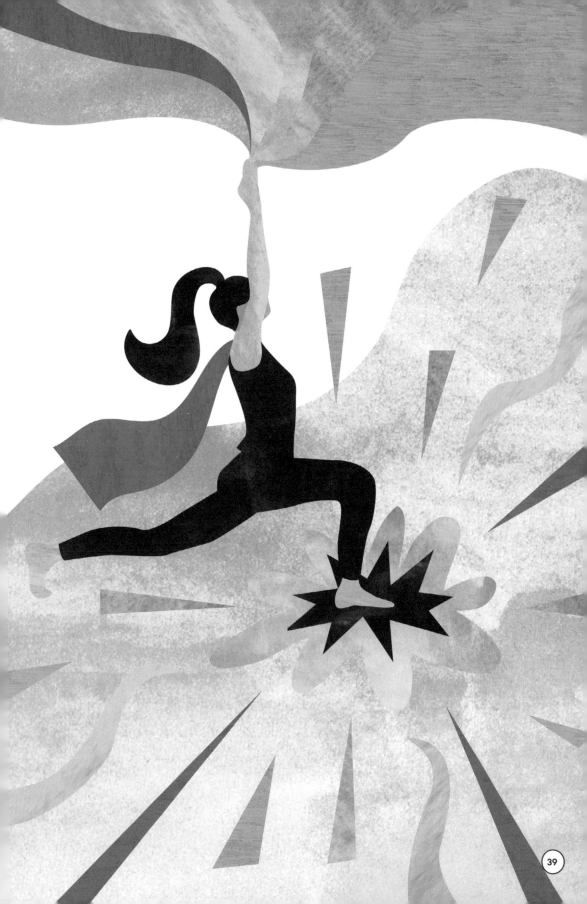

WARRIOR II ● ● ·

Virabhadrasana II

Warrior II is a powerful pose that strengthens the muscles of the thighs, buttocks, chest and arms. It also opens the chest and shoulders, which can help to increase breathing capacity and boost circulation. Practice of Warrior II helps to nurture a strong connection to your inner strength and wisdom while encouraging the gaze and intention towards achieving your goals.

Here's how to explore the pose:

1. Stand in Mountain pose (page 22), facing towards the long edge of your mat. Take a few deep breaths, bring your thoughts within and connect to your inner strength and wisdom.

2. On an out-breath, step your feet wide apart to a point that is comfortable. Raise your arms so they come level with the shoulders (try to position your ankles below your wrists). Keep the arms parallel to the floor, palms facing downwards, and toes facing the long edge of your mat. Take a few deep breaths.

3. Turn your right foot out 90 degrees from your body and your left foot to an angle of around 15 degrees. The heels of the feet should be aligned.

4. On an out-breath, lower your hips, forming a right angle with your right leg – the right knee should be lined up above your ankle, but not beyond it. Your thigh is parallel to the floor and the shin is vertical to the floor.

5. Keep your left leg straight. If you feel a little unstable, try to think about pressing down the outer edge of the left foot.

6. Focus on opening your chest by lifting the front of your torso upwards. Push the fingertips of both hands away from you.

7. Turn your head and upper torso to face the direction of your bent right leg and outstretched right arm and hand. Continue stretching into the fingertips of both hands, which will help to maintain a straight torso.

8. Focus your gaze in the direction of your right hand. Take a few deep breaths, feeling strong in mind and body. You may also choose to focus your mind and intention on a goal you'd like to achieve.

9. To come out of the pose, on an in-breath, push down through your left leg and slowly straighten your right leg. Now, turn your feet, chest and hips back to a forwards-facing position. Step your feet back together and lower your arms alongside your body once more. Take a few breaths. Observe how you feel. When ready, repeat the sequence, leading with your left leg.

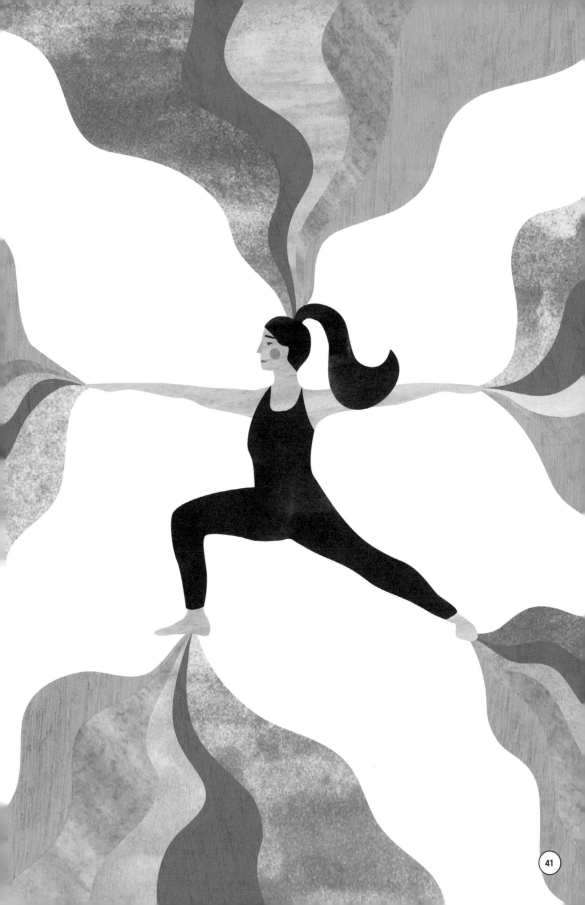

WARRIOR III

Virabhadrasana III

A combination of lightness of being and physical strength, Warrior III is the most challenging of the Warrior poses. It's great for the legs, arms and torso, while improving balance, posture, coordination and concentration.

Here's how to explore the pose:

1. Stand tall, legs hip-width apart. Place your hands at heart centre in Prayer pose (Step 6, page 21). Take a moment to breathe, calm your mind and connect with your strength within.

2. On an in-breath, take your left foot back, so your feet are about a metre apart – or to a point that's comfortable. Bending the right leg, lower your hips, keeping the torso upright, so it forms a right angle with your right leg in a lunge position. Raise your hands skywards above the head in Prayer pose or with fingers interlaced, index fingers touching and pointing upwards.

3. On an out-breath, ground your right foot, tense the muscles in your right leg and keep your hips level. Engage your core by drawing the stomach muscles towards your spine (this will help to protect your back). Extend the torso upwards and flow forwards from your hips, extending through the crown of the head and arms, which are still outstretched, to a position that's parallel to the ground. At the same time, raise the left leg, lengthening backwards through the soles. The hips face the floor.

4. Come to a position where the torso and left leg are lined up parallel to the ground, with your right leg straight and grounded. Take a few breaths here. Breathe in a lightness of being and strength within as you float in Warrior III.

5. To come out of the pose, on an in-breath, slowly lower the left leg to the ground. Moving from your hips, raise your torso back to standing, lowering the arms to your sides.

6. Take a few breaths. Observe the effect of the pose on your being. When ready, repeat on the opposite side, stepping back with your right leg.

Tips:

✳ If you feel a bit wobbly, try resting your hands on a ledge that's at a similar height to your outstretched arms, so you're not leaning down.

✳ You could also rest your extended back foot on the back of a securely positioned chair.

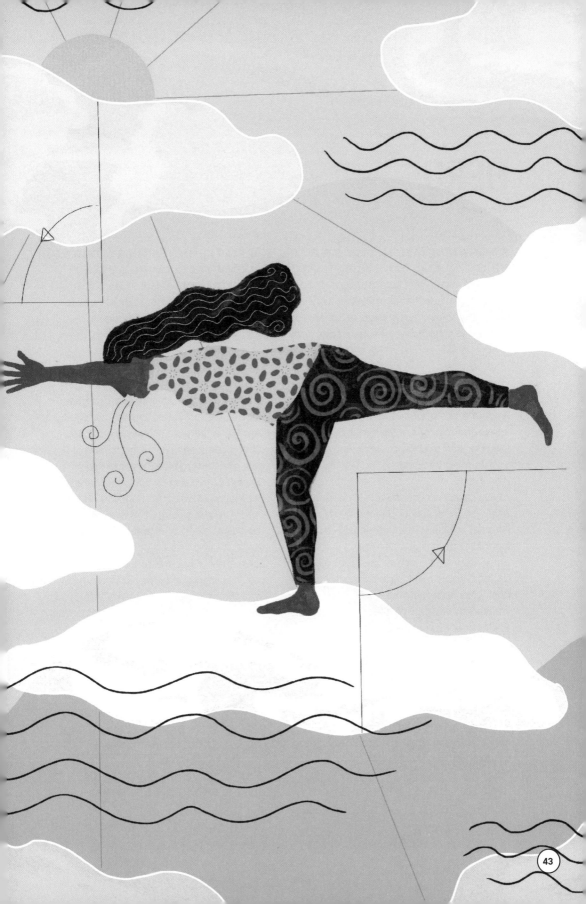

HERO

Virasana

A seated pose that will help you to hold your head up high and find the strength within, Hero can be used for meditation and breathing exercises. As well as strengthening the quadriceps, it works the muscles around the ankles, aids spine alignment and posture, and builds flexibility in the knees, ankles and thighs. Anyone with knee or ankle injuries is advised to avoid this pose, as are those who have a heart condition.

Here's how to explore the pose:

1. Start in an upright kneeling position on your mat. Keep your hips over your knees and the tops of your feet flat on the mat, with toes pressing downwards and pointing backwards.

2. Open a space between your shins by moving your ankles and feet slightly apart, keeping your knees together. Lower your buttocks into the gap between your feet until you're sitting on the mat. A block or folded blanket can be placed under the buttocks if that feels more comfortable – a blanket can also be placed under the ankles or knees for support.

3. On an in-breath, extend your spine upwards from your tailbone, engage your core, drawing your belly towards your spine. Hold your head high, face forwards. Release your shoulders away from your ears and lift and roll your shoulder blades towards each other at the back.

4. When comfortable, gently rest your hands on your knees. You could also practise a *mudra* – a Sanskrit word, it means 'seal', 'gesture' or 'mark', and describes a symbolic hand gesture, used in Hindu and Buddhist practices. For this pose, you might choose *Gyan mudra*, where you gently bring together the tips of the thumb and index finger on each hand (the other fingers remain open and softly stretched apart, with the palms opening upwards). Breathe here for a few comfortable breaths (or longer if preferred). If you experience pain, carefully come out of the pose (see below).

5. To come out of the pose, press your palms into the ground, lift your buttocks, bring your ankles together and move your buttocks over your feet to come to a sitting position on the ground. Slowly straighten both legs in front of you and relax.

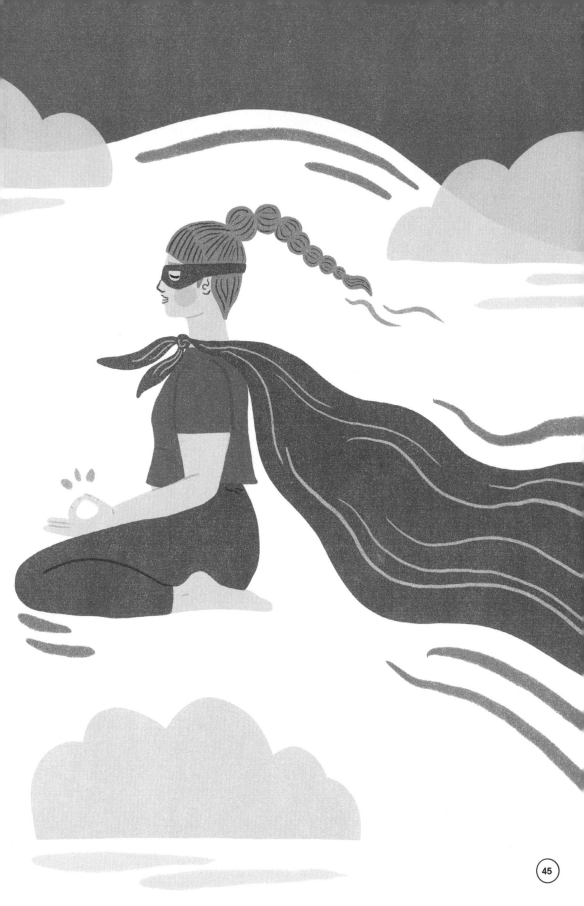

BUTTERFLY

Baddha konasana

Butterflies are a beautiful, colourful reminder of the world's magic and miracles – research has shown they can even remember things learned in their caterpillar stage. Like the butterfly, people are constantly growing, developing and transforming into a greater version of themselves. Butterfly pose provides a lovely space to connect with your beautiful self. It strengthens and opens the hip area and stimulates energy flow to the lower abdomen, easing cramps and discomfort and soothing the lower back.

Here's how to explore the pose:

1. Sit on the floor, legs outstretched. Hold the spine upright, tall and straight. Take a few gentle breaths to settle your mind and body.

2. On an out-breath, bend the knees and draw the feet towards the groin, bringing together the soles so they face each other. Gently wrap the hands around the feet, ankles or shins. Allow the inner thighs to relax and let the knees open downwards, towards the floor, as far as is comfortable.

3. Sitting up tall, broaden and lift the chest. Take a few deep breaths in this position and allow yourself to observe fully how you feel.

4. On an out-breath, fold the upper torso forwards from the hips. If you can, rest the head on the soles of the feet. If not, fold forwards as far as is comfortable. Take a few breaths, then lift the body back to sitting tall.

5. Observe if your practice has helped to release tension in the lower back and made you feel more calm and relaxed.

Tip:

* If you'd like to vary the pose, while sitting up tall at Step 3, move the knees gently up and down – a little like a butterfly flapping its wings.

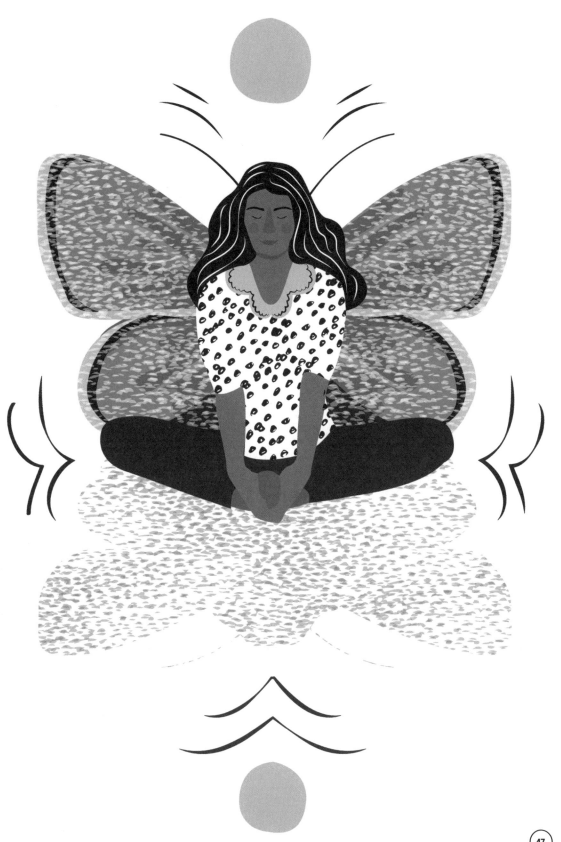

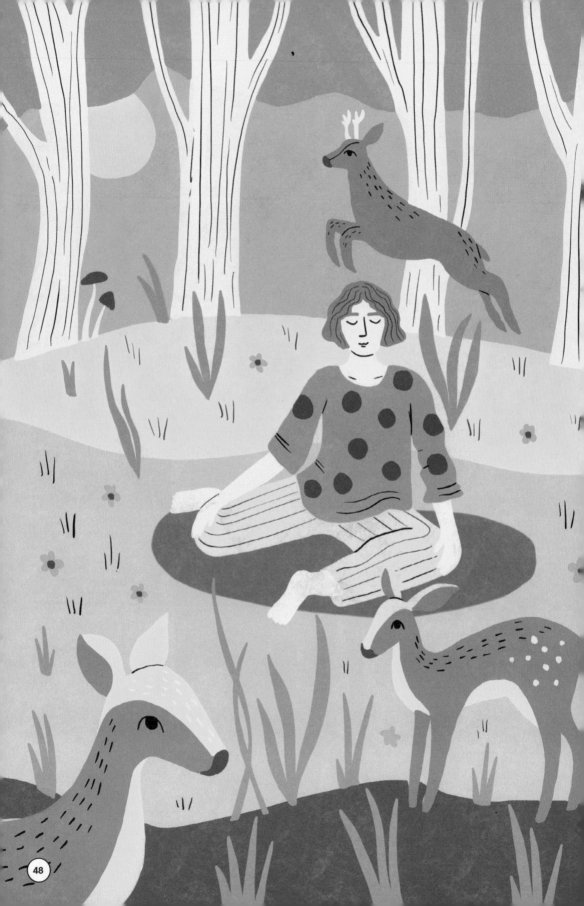

DEER

Mrigasana

The deer roams forests, woods and grasslands and is known for its instincts, speed, agility and grace. Deer pose is a gentle seated twist that works the hip flexors, knees, quadriceps, lower back and glutes. It improves digestion and helps bring harmony to the mind.

Here's how to explore the pose:

1. Begin in an upright seated position, with the soles of the feet together and the knees opening outwards, as in Butterfly (page 46).

2. On an in-breath, gently open the hips, take the right leg behind your body, with the knee remaining bent at a 90-degree angle. If this feels painful, adjust until it feels comfortable. The left leg remains in front of you with the knee bent – also at a 90-degree angle. (The hips remain in contact with the ground, but if you find there's a gap, try sitting on a folded blanket or yoga block.)

3. To add a fold to the pose, on an in-breath, grow tall through the spine, gently rotate the upper torso from the hips towards the left and, as you exhale, bear down to the left and bring your hands to rest on the ground outside your left thigh.

4. If you're comfortable to take the stretch further, lower your upper torso and rest on your elbows, with your forearms and hands flat on the ground, your head folded forwards or resting on the ground between your arms. Whichever position you're in, take a few comfortable breaths.

5. To come out of the pose, lean away from the back right foot, then bring your right leg back around in front of you and return to Butterfly, with the soles of the feet touching.

6. Take a few breaths here before repeating the sequence, this time taking the left leg behind.

CHURNING THE MILL

Chakki chalanasana

The phrase Churning the mill comes from the movement used to grind wheat with a traditional hand-operated grain mill, commonly used in Indian villages. This pose works the chest and abdominal muscles, tones the arms and legs, and strengthens the hip region. It also improves digestion. As with the axle of a wheel, the circular motion around the base of the spine results in an increase in energy, which flows up the back.

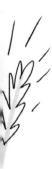

Here's how to explore the pose:

1. Sit upright with your back straight and tall, your hips flat and square on the mat and your legs extended in front of you. Keeping your back straight and your head high, face forwards. Take a few breaths, ground and centre your mind and body.

2. On an in-breath, gently push your legs apart to a position that's comfortable, keeping them flat on the ground.

3. On another in-breath, raise your arms to shoulder height, stretching them out in front of you. Join your palms together and interlock your fingers (palms facing towards you).

4. Again, on an in-breath, flow forwards from your waist extending your interlocked arms over your right leg, parallel to the ground, reaching towards your right foot. Then flow them across to your left foot.

5. As you breathe out, circle your arms to your chest, leaning your upper torso backwards from the waist, then come back round to the right foot. Breathe in here and continue in an anticlockwise direction, moving from the waist. Remember to maintain a straight back, arms and legs as you circle your upper torso round.

6. Continue for five or 10 rotations anticlockwise, then repeat for five or 10 rotations clockwise.

7. Come to stillness. Check your position is once more upright, release your hands and then lie back on the floor and enjoy a few moments of peace.

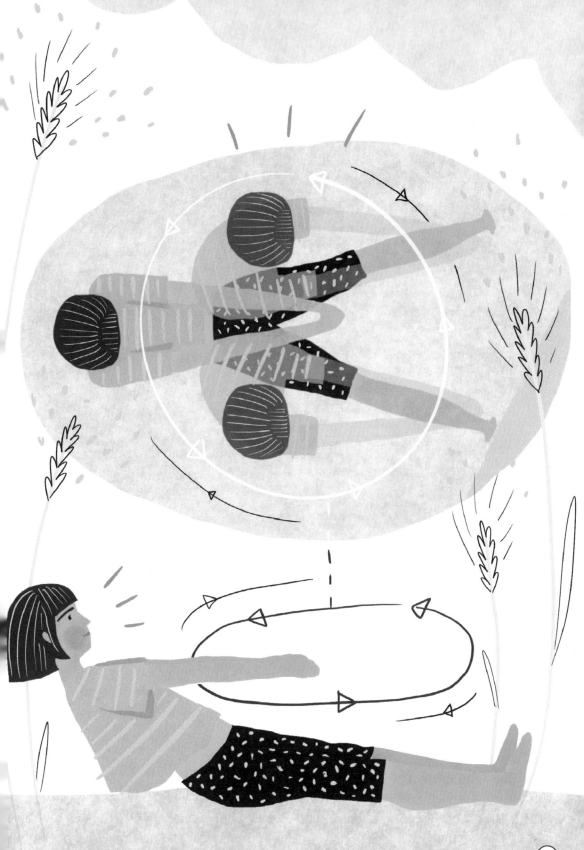

SITTING FORWARD BEND

Paschimottanasana

A pose that helps to release internal tension is Sitting forward bend. As with Standing forward bend (page 24), it lengthens the hamstrings and stretches the back, easing compression and tension in the vertebrae and helping to calm racing thoughts.

Here's how to explore the pose:

1. Sit on the floor, legs stretched out straight in front of you with your heels pushing forwards and toes heading skywards. With your hands resting on the floor beside your hips, take a few deep breaths and observe how your body feels.

2. On an in-breath, raise your arms above your head and, lifting from your tailbone, lift your upper torso skywards.

3. On an out-breath, fold forwards from your hips, extending a straight spine forwards towards your feet. Bring your upper torso towards the tops of your legs and slowly continue stretching forwards (making sure to keep a straight back) until your head is the last thing to touch down. Your hands are gently wrapped around your feet or ankles. (It can be difficult to fully release over your legs, so only reach forwards to a point that's comfortable. It shouldn't be painful. With practice, your extension forwards will increase, and you will be able to release a little further.)

4. Come out of the pose on an in-breath. From your hips, slowly raise your torso back up to a seated position, vertebrae by vertebrae, with your head coming up last and your arms flowing back up and round to rest alongside your body.

5. Take a few deep breaths here and observe how your body feels. Notice if you are experiencing less tension and feel more relaxed in your being.

Tip:

* Many practitioners find it challenging to reach their toes in Sitting forward bend. Another option at Step 3 is to loop a yoga belt around the soles of your feet and lower yourself, with a flat back, to a point that's comfortable.

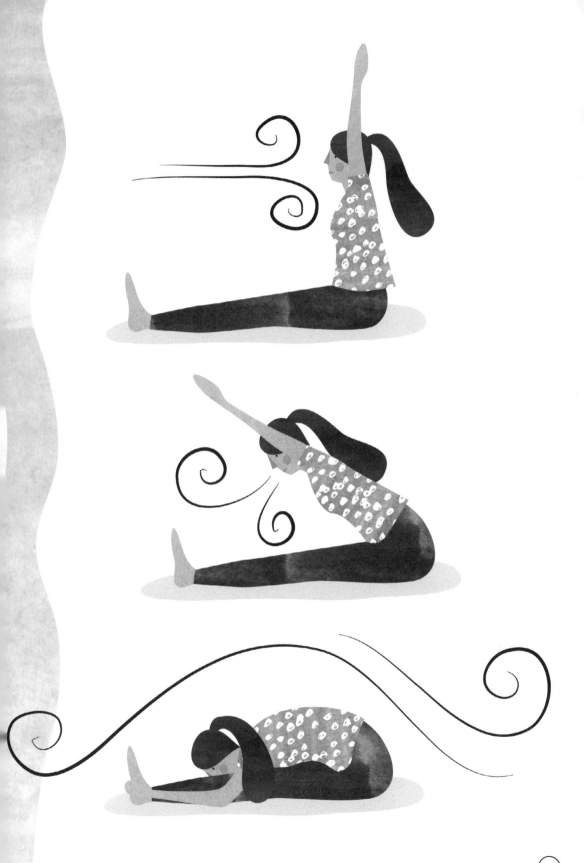

SHOELACE

Padukabandhini asana

Shoelace pose is named for the way the legs loop and bend around each other as laces do when you tie a bow (*Paduka* meaning 'footwear' in Sanskrit and *bandhini* meaning 'lace'). This pose supports hip mobility, works the muscles in the lower back, glutes and legs, and stimulates the gallbladder and kidneys. It's also said to calm the mind.

Here's how to explore the pose:

1. Sit upright with your back straight and tall, your hips flat and square on the mat and your legs extended in front of you.

2. On an in-breath, bend your left knee, draw your foot towards you, lift it over your right leg and bring your left heel to touch the ground on the outside of your right hip.

3. On another in-breath, bend your right knee, sliding your heel to the outside of your left hip. Your left knee is stacked above your right knee – position them centrally between your hips. (If this is painful or uncomfortable, leave the right leg extended.)

4. Breathe here. Extend your spine upwards, face forwards, chest open, arms flowing alongside your torso as you gently hold your feet. Take a few breaths here. Yoga blocks, bolsters or folded blankets can be used as needed.

5. If you'd like to, you can add an optional forward fold here. Lower the upper torso from the hips so that your heart is over your interlaced legs. Use your arms to support your weight by resting your hands on the ground or on a yoga block. Hold for a few comfortable breaths.

6. When ready to come out of the pose, press through your hands and slowly roll up through your spine to an upright position. Place your hands slightly behind you, lean back and release your legs back to the original position extended on the ground in front of you. Repeat on the opposite side.

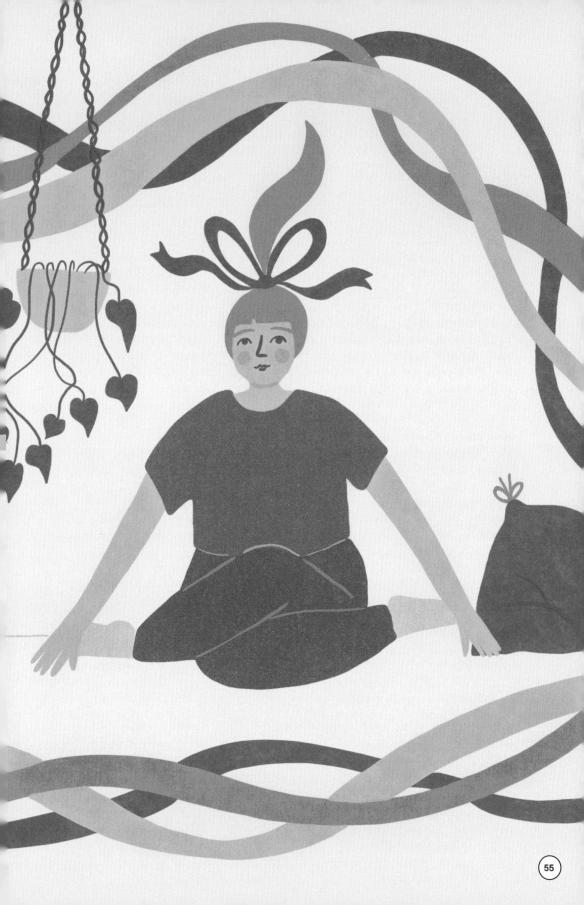

LOTUS

Padmasana

The lotus flower is a symbol of purity, enlightenment, self-regeneration and rebirth. And, believe it or not, it blooms most beautifully from the deepest and thickest mud. Practising Lotus is said to calm the mind and prepare you for deep meditation. Lotus is an advanced posture, however, so make sure to allow your body to open and blossom at its own comfortable pace. Follow the directions carefully and ease yourself into this pose slowly, making sure to fully warm up first. Anyone with knee, ankle or hip injuries is advised to avoid this pose, as are those with chronic inflammation of the joints or those who need to be careful of their blood circulation. Be gentle on your being.

Here's how to explore the pose:

1. Sit tall on the floor with your legs extended out in front of you.

2. Bend your right knee, rotate it outwards from your hips, while at the same time rolling your left thigh open. Bring your right ankle to rest on the crease of your left hip, with the soles of the feet upwards.

3. Bend your left knee, bring it towards you and slide it up over your right leg to rest with the soles upwards. The tops of your feet and ankle should be resting on your hip crease.

4. Ground into your sitting bones. Now, breathing in, raise and open your chest.

Gently rest your hands on your knees or in a *mudra*. A popular one used in meditation is *Gyan* (Step 4, page 44).

5. Sit and breathe here for as long as you wish and you find comfortable. To release the pose, gently extend both legs, one at a time, along the floor in front of you. Repeat the pose, beginning with the left ankle in the right hip crease.

6. Lotus is a seat for meditation. If used regularly, it's important to remember to alternate the cross of the leg daily.

Tip:

* Don't be disheartened if full Lotus is too uncomfortable to practise. Everyone's body is different. An alternative is Easy pose – *Sukhasana* in Sanskrit – which is any comfortable, cross-legged seated position.

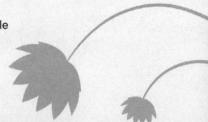

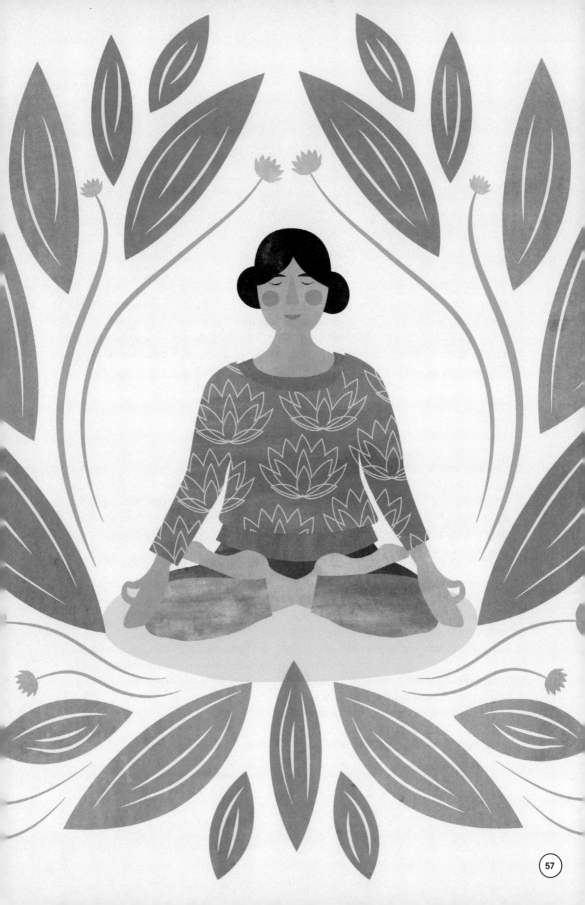

BOAT

Navasana

As you go through life, the waves go up and down, sometimes they're calm, occasionally they're choppy. Boat pose builds strength within, which will help you to surf the waves, whatever their size. This strong pose engages with the core to create physical and mental strength, tone stomach muscles, strengthen the lower back and encourage a healthy metabolism. It also nurtures an ability to conquer tricky situations, resulting in increased confidence and an improved sense of self. Anyone who has a neck injury or who experiences headaches or low blood pressure is advised not to practise Boat pose.

Here's how to explore the pose:

1. Sit on the floor with your legs straight in front of you and your torso upright and strong. Lift from the tailbone and open the chest by bringing the shoulders down and back.

2. Press your hands to the floor, a little behind your hips with your fingers pointing towards your feet. Sit tall as you slowly lean back. Take a few breaths here as you find your point of balance on your sit bones.

3. On an out-breath, bend your knees and lift your feet off the floor. Engaging your core and stomach muscles, point your legs and feet upwards towards the sky at an angle that feels comfortable for you.

4. Keeping your arms straight, stretch them out parallel to the floor, holding them on the outside of your legs with your fingers pointing forwards.

5. Take a few steady in- and out-breaths, holding the pose for a few seconds, as long as it feels comfortable to do so. Do not place strain on your back.

6. To come out of the pose, on an out-breath, slowly lower your legs to the floor and, on an in-breath, sit back upright.

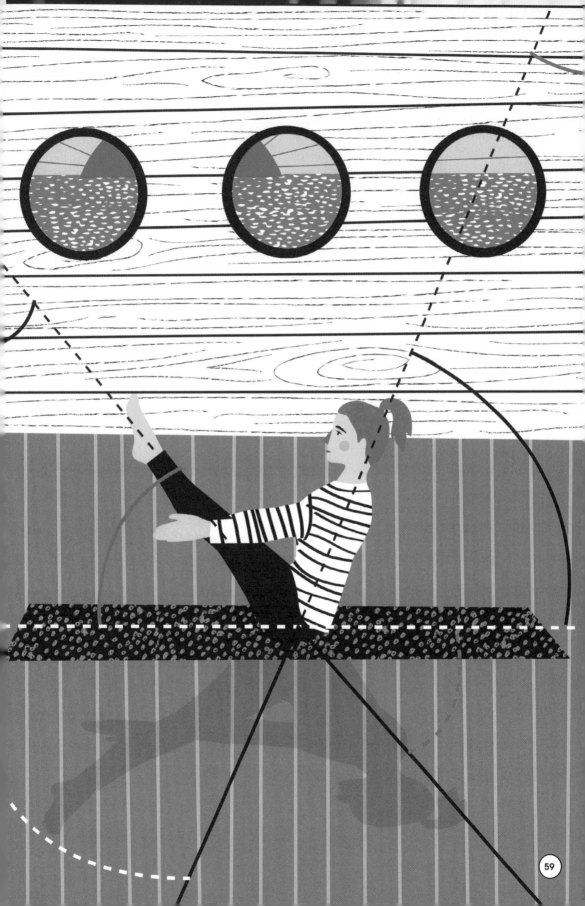

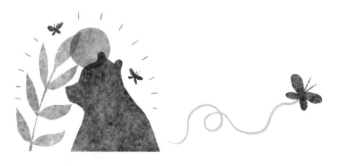

BALANCING BEAR

Merudandasana

Bears are strong, beautiful creatures who live in harmony with their environment. Balancing bear pose helps to improve balance, focus and concentration, while strengthening your core and spine. It also supports your digestive system and stretches your hips and hamstrings.

Here's how to explore the pose:

1. Begin in a seated position, with the soles of your feet together and your knees dropping towards the ground as in Butterfly (page 46). Take a few breaths here, to ground and focus your being.

2. Holding each big toe between your index finger, middle finger and thumb, direct your gaze to a fixed point in front of you.

3. Ground down through your sit bones, then, engaging your core muscles, draw your navel towards your spine. Keeping your back long, lean back slightly from the hips, balancing on your coccyx (a small bone at the base of your spine).

4. On an in-breath, engage the muscles in your legs, core and arms. Then, holding on to your big toes, extend your legs outwards and upwards, to a comfortable height and angle. If you're struggling to fully extend your legs, it's OK to slightly bend your knees. With practice, you may be able to slowly work your way up to

a fully extended leg position, but only ever stretch as far as is comfortable.

5. Balance and breathe here. Take a moment to enjoy the pose.

6. On an out-breath, release by bending your knees and bringing your feet back to the ground in front of you. Return your torso to an upright seated position.

7. Extend your legs out in front of you and give them a little shake to release any tension.

8. Sit here for a moment, breathing steadily. You might also choose to lie flat on the ground with arms and legs extended in Corpse pose (page 114) for a few moments.

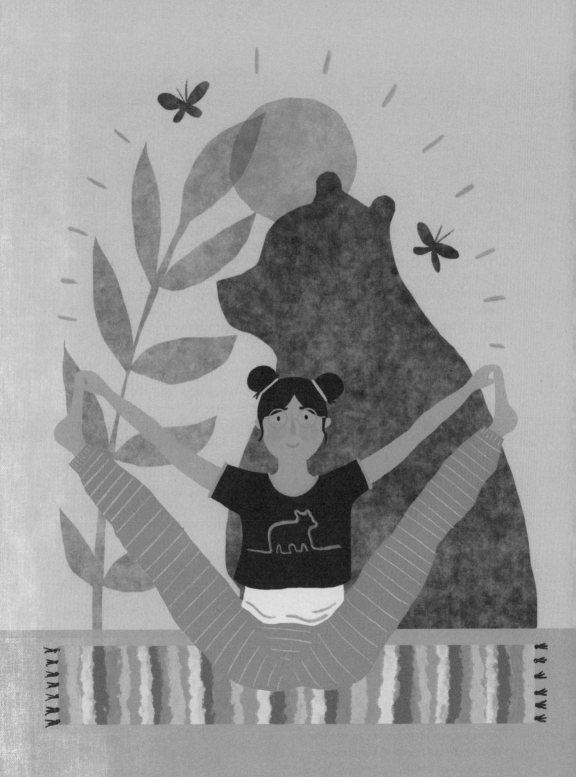

CAT

Marjaryasana

Cat is a simple yet dynamic pose that harnesses the power, strength and agility of our feline friends. Ancient Egyptians believed cats had divine energy, which may be the reason they're said to have nine lives. The key body part worked here is the spine. This plays an important role in the health of the body by housing the spinal cord – a column of nerves connecting your brain to the rest of your body. Maintaining its strength and flexibility benefits your whole being. Cat pose is often practised as a flow with Cow pose (page 64).

Here's how to explore the pose:

1. Warm up the wrists by gently rotating them clockwise and anticlockwise.

2. Come to all fours on your mat. Align your arms and wrists with your shoulder sockets and place your palms flat on the floor with fingers gently splayed. Position your knees below your hips, shins resting on the floor, with the tops of your feet flat, soles facing skywards (you may wish to place a folded blanket under your knees). With a flat back and your head and neck in line, extend forwards, gazing to the ground. This is often referred to as neutral or tabletop position.

3. Pushing downwards through the arms and legs, on an out-breath, draw your tummy in and round your spine skywards by releasing the crown of the head and tailbone towards the mat (think of a soft convex shape). Keep pushing into the floor with your hands to help broaden the shoulder blades, and keep your head and neck relaxed. Your gaze is directed towards your tummy.

4. Breathing in and out, gently explore this stretch of the spine, and try flowing through into the concave shape of Cow pose (page 64, overleaf) then back into Cat a few times.

5. To come out of the pose, walk your hands back to kneeling, gently roll out your wrists and enjoy a moment's stillness.

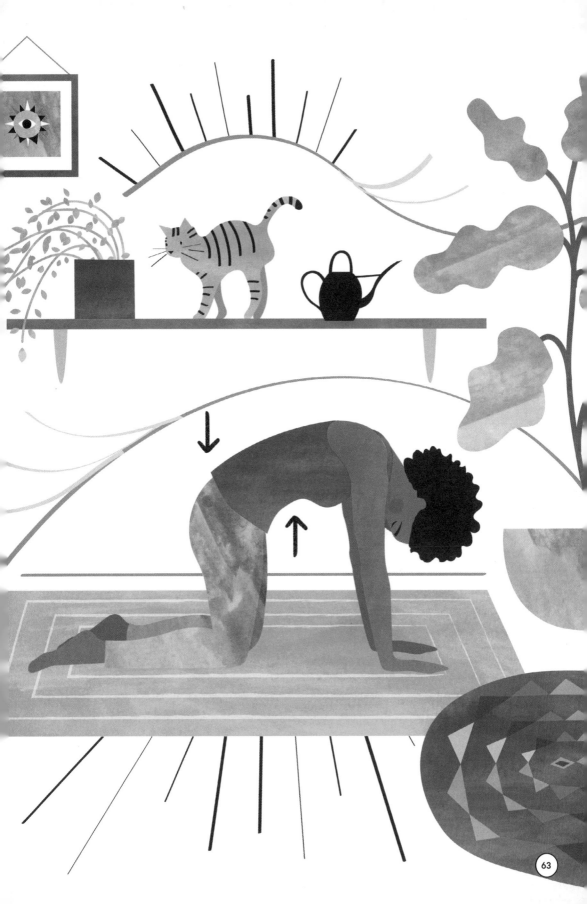

COW

Bitilasana

Cows have sacred status in several religions, including Hinduism, Jainism and Buddhism, and are revered in many cultures as a symbol of fertility, generosity, motherhood and prosperity. Cow pose works the spine, strengthens and stretches the muscles in the back, abdomen, shoulders and hips, and helps release tension. It also provides a gentle warm-up and is often paired with Cat pose (page 62) ahead of more advanced back bends and flow sequences.

Here's how to explore the pose:

1. Warm up the wrists by gently rotating them clockwise and anticlockwise.

2. Begin on all fours in tabletop position (Step 2, page 62).

3. On an out-breath, lift and roll your shoulders back and, opening your chest, gently extend your neck forwards and chin upwards. At the same time, lower your tummy towards the ground. Stretch all the way along your spine, from the base of the skull to your tailbone.

4. As your spine curves downwards, tilt your pelvis, so that your tailbone extends upwards and backwards. Keep the back of your neck long and engage the abdominals by drawing your navel towards your spine.

5. Exhale and return your body to the neutral tabletop position or Cat (page 62). If you find it's hard on your knees, place a folded blanket underneath them to provide cushioning.

6. Breathing in and out, gently explore this stretch of the spine, either flowing through into Cat or returning to tabletop, whichever is preferred.

7. When you feel ready, bring your body to a kneeling position. You may also choose to fold forwards and rest for a few moments in Child's pose (page 108), with your forehead on the mat and your arms resting along the outside of the legs, palms facing upwards.

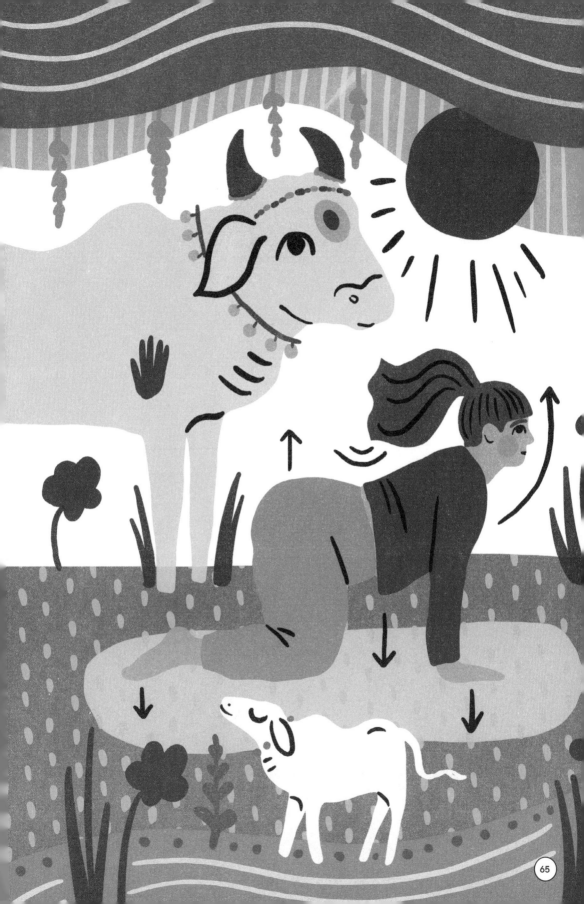

HAPPY BABY

Ananda balasana

Babies are flexible, freely expressive of their emotions and share love unconditionally. Happy baby is a gentle, playful pose that can be enjoyed by all levels of practitioner. It has many benefits, easing tension in the lower back, stretching the hips and thighs, and calming the mind. It also helps to release stress and fatigue. Best of all, it rarely fails to raise a smile. Anyone who has neck or knee injuries is advised not to practise this pose.

Here's how to explore the pose:

1. Begin by lying flat on your back on your yoga mat, legs outstretched, feet facing upwards. Breathe here for a moment. Connect with the youngest version of yourself that you can think back to – perhaps you can remember being a toddler, or even younger.

2. On an out-breath, bend your knees, slowly bringing them towards your chest, with the soles of your feet flat and facing the ceiling.

3. Take hold of the outside of your feet with your hands. If that's difficult, loop a yoga strap around the sole of each foot – or hold onto your ankles or shins instead.

4. Spread your knees apart to a position that's slightly wider than your torso, then move them gently towards your armpits. Position your ankles above your knees, with the soles of the feet facing the ceiling. Breathe here.

5. The head, neck, shoulders, back and hips remain flat on the ground, opening and releasing downwards. Relax the face and gently rock from side to side like a happy baby.

6. When ready, release your feet and lower your legs back to the ground. Gently bring yourself up to a comfortable cross-legged seated position.

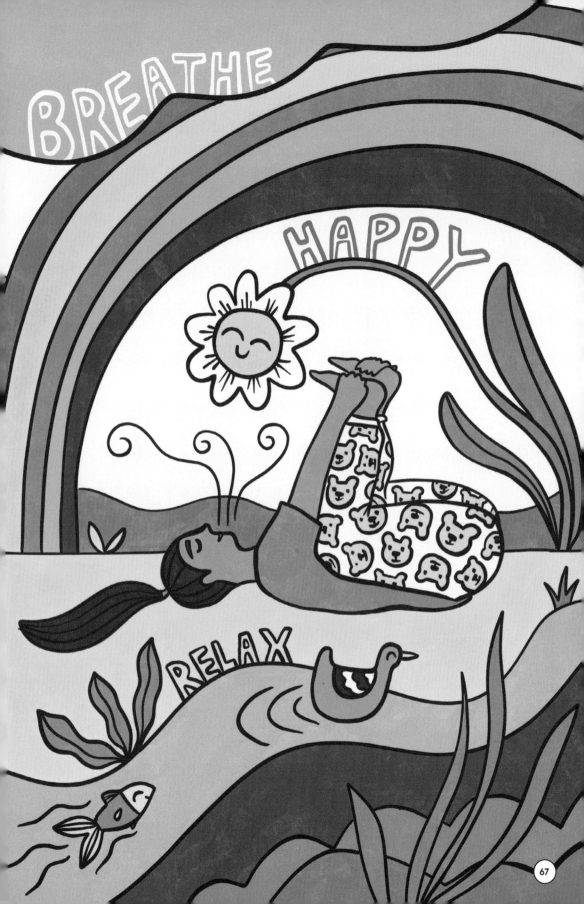

RECLINING BUTTERFLY

Supta baddha konasana

Just watching these graceful insects is relaxing, so it's perhaps no surprise that practising Reclining butterfly also releases tension and stress in the body, while helping to restore calm. It improves flexibility in the hips and thighs, circulation in the abdomen and pelvic area, and supports the elimination of waste energy. The chest area also gently opens and releases tension in the upper torso, neck, head and arms. Ease yourself into this pose slowly and carefully.

Here's how to explore the pose:

1. Sit upright with your back straight and tall, your hips flat and square on the mat and your legs extended in front of you. Take a few breaths here to calm your centre and focus your being.

2. On an in-breath, bend your knees, drawing your feet towards your pelvic area, as close as is comfortably possible (don't overstretch). Bring the soles of your feet together and allow your knees and thighs to open out to rest gently on the floor – or as close to it as is comfortable.

3. From here, bring your hands down to rest on the floor beside your hips. Then, with the assistance of your arms, gently lower your upper body to the floor. If it feels uncomfortable or painful at any time, don't push it, stay in the upright seated position and just breathe, making the most of the stillness.

4. The arms can be released away from the torso, palms opening upwards, or placed on the stomach area.

5. Relax, release and breathe. Remain in this position for a few minutes or as long as feels comfortable and you would like to enjoy the benefits of the pose.

6. To come out of the pose, release your legs, turn on your side and gently bring your torso back to sitting with the assistance of your arms.

Tip:

∗ Use yoga blocks, cushions or blankets to support your knees and back in this pose and make it as comfortable as possible to surrender to its benefits.

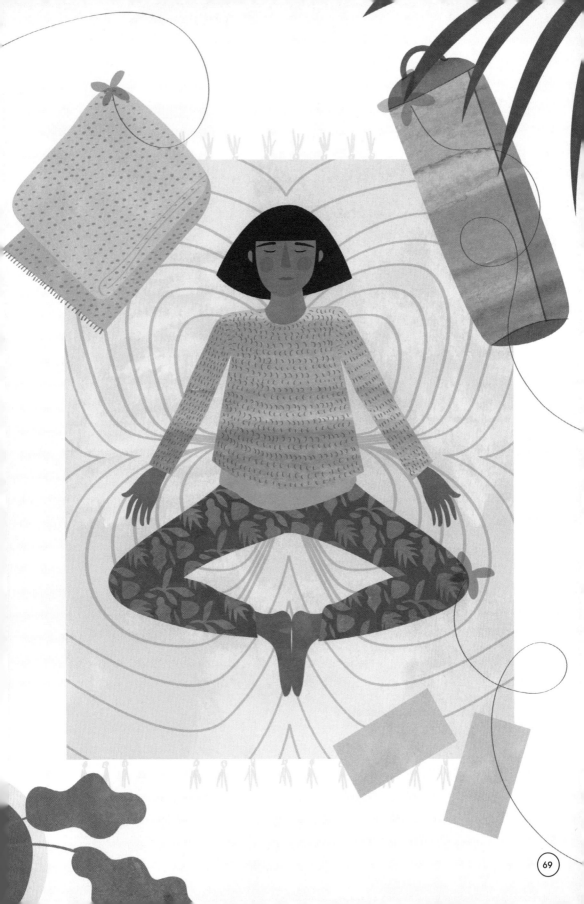

RECLINING HAND-TO-BIG-TOE

Supta padangusthasana

Lie down and release with Reclining hand-to-big-toe pose. This powerful stretch helps to relieve lower back pain, stimulates flow in the lower abdominal region, releases tension in the hamstrings and calves, strengthens knee and leg muscles and helps to calm the mind.

Here's how to get into the pose:

1. To begin, lie flat on the ground, facing upwards, legs strongly extended from hip to heel, with the feet flexed and the torso opening and releasing to the ground. Breathe here for a moment.

2. On an in-breath, bend your right knee and draw it to your chest, giving it a little hug. Then either take hold of the big toe on your right foot with your thumb and first two fingers, or loop your yoga strap around the sole of the right foot, holding the strap with both hands.

3. Slowly straighten your right leg and extend it from the hip upwards, pushing the heel towards the ceiling. At this point, your arms will be fully extended as you hold either your big toe or the strap.

4. The left foot, leg, both hips and torso stay strong on the floor, opening and releasing to the ground.

5. Keep the muscles of both legs active by extending through the heels. To avoid locking the knees, engage the thighs and lift the kneecaps.

6. If it's comfortable, you can increase the stretch in the back of the leg by drawing the right foot a little closer towards your head. Breathe here for a few minutes.

7. From this point, you have the option of turning the right leg outwards from the hip (so the kneecap and toes look to the right) before slowly moving the whole leg out to the right. Hold it at a comfortable height off the ground. Breathe here for a few moments.

8. Gently return the right leg to the upright position. Release the strap or big toe, breathe and lower your leg slowly back down to the ground.

9. Rest here for a moment, then repeat, leading with the left leg.

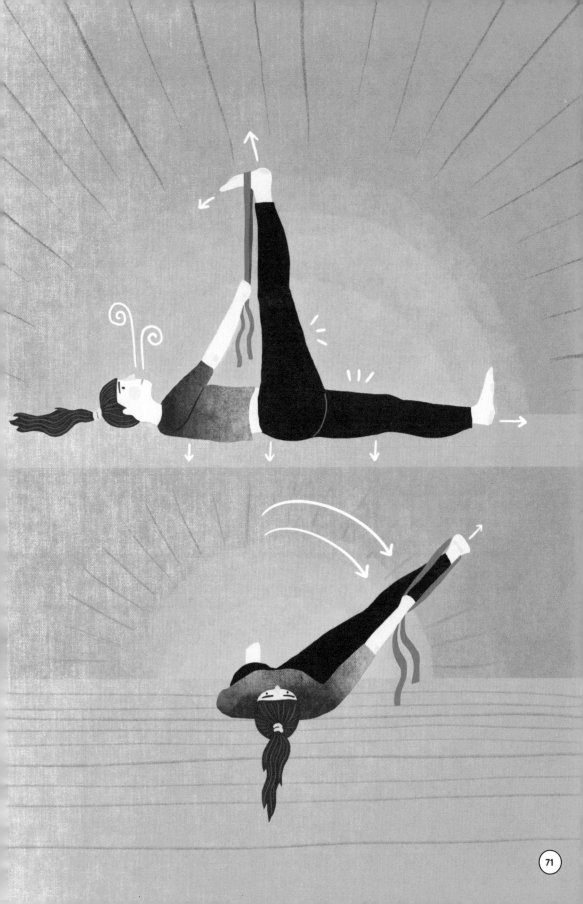

DOWNWARD-FACING DOG

Adho mukha svanasana

Friendly, playful, loyal, full of energy – it's no surprise dogs are often one of the best-loved members of the family. And one of the most popular yoga poses also has a canine reference, Downward-facing dog. This much-practised pose lengthens and stretches the spine, releases tension in the upper torso, legs and arms, and provides an oxygen boost to the body. It also builds strength in the arms, shoulders, wrists, abdominals and legs. Another benefit is that it stimulates the nervous system, improving memory and concentration.

Here's how to explore the pose:

1. Warm up the wrists by gently rotating them clockwise and anticlockwise.

2. Begin on all fours in tabletop position (Step 2, page 62).

3. From this position, turn your toes under. Then, on an out-breath, pushing downwards evenly through your arms and legs, raise your hips skywards. Engage your stomach muscles by drawing the navel back towards the spine.

4. Your body will form a triangle shape. There will be two straight lines. The first flows down from your hips along your spine through your arms and then into your hands on the floor. The second flows from your hips along the full length of your legs and into the feet.

5. Stretch into the legs, lowering the heels towards the floor (be careful not to lock out the knees). If possible, place the feet flat on the floor, but this isn't essential. It's better to bend the knees slightly and maintain a straight back. Be careful not to overstretch to the point of discomfort or pain.

6. Hang your head carefully and gently between your arms (you should be able to see your tummy). Roll the shoulders back and down and keep the hips lifted.

7. Take a few deep breaths in this position, feeling the lovely stretch in your hamstrings, back, spine and arms, and enjoying the release in the neck.

8. When you're ready, bend your knees towards the floor, returning to tabletop. From here, walk your hands back to a seated kneeling position and roll out your wrists to release any tension.

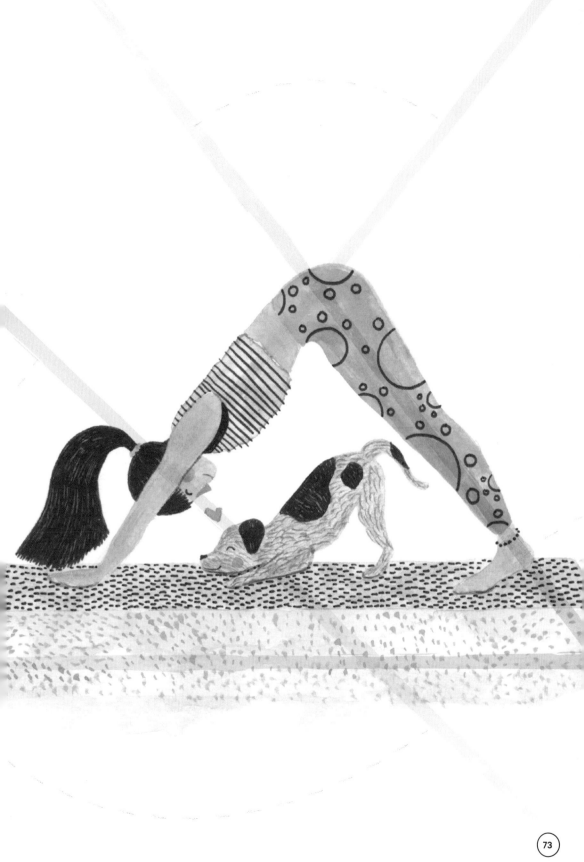

PLANK

Phalakasana

Plank pose has many physical and mental benefits. It tones the abdominal, chest and lower-body muscles, while strengthening the arms, spine, legs and solar plexus (a collection of nerves in the abdomen). It also helps to build mental resilience and can increase willpower, focus and direction.

Here's how to explore the pose:

1. Begin on all fours in tabletop position. (Step 2, page 62). Focus on pressing through your index fingers and thumbs and keeping the shoulders open.

2. Take a few breaths, engaging your core stomach muscles and channelling your inner mental focus.

3. On an out-breath, tuck your toes under. Step your right foot straight back, followed by your left foot. Lift the hips, thighs and abdomen so that your body forms a straight line. Keep your shoulders strong and open. The crown of your head extends forwards, keeping total alignment.

4. Maintain the pose by pushing downwards through your arms and backwards and downwards through your feet. Keep the stomach muscles engaged, drawing your navel towards your spine and extending your tailbone towards your feet.

5. Take a few breaths here and observe and feel the flow of strength within.

6. To come out of the pose, slowly lower your knees to the floor and walk your hands back to a kneeling position. You may also wish to roll out the wrists and rest in Child's pose (page 108) to release the shoulders and back.

Tip:

* Another option at Step 3 is to bring your knees down to the floor, while maintaining the stretch and incline on the torso.

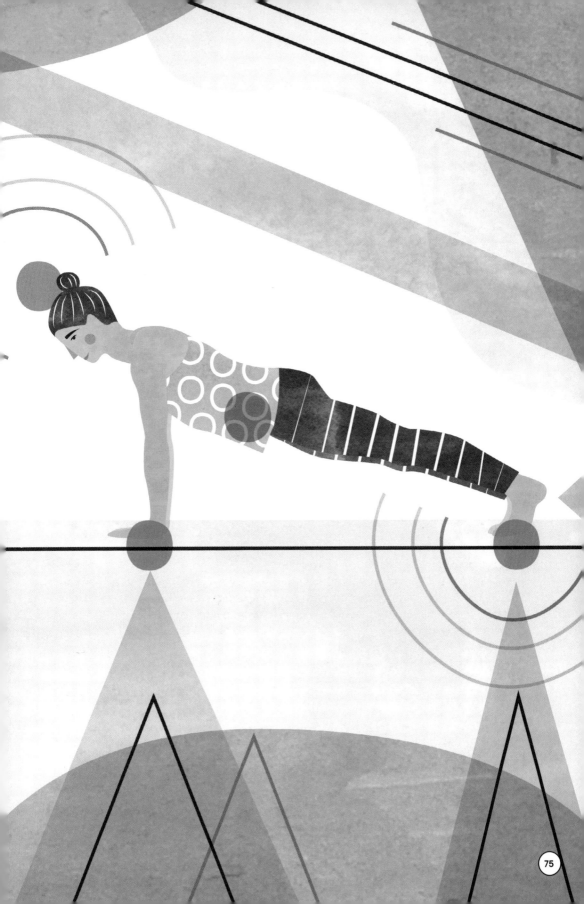

HALF LORD OF THE FISHES

Ardha matsyendrasana

Twisting postures increase suppleness in your spine, stimulate internal organs – particularly your kidneys, stomach, pancreas and spleen – and stretch the back, shoulders and neck. Half lord of the fishes is a gentle variation of a seated twist.

Here's how to explore the pose:

1. Sit on the floor, legs stretched out straight in front of you with your heels pushing forwards and toes skywards. Take a few breaths to centre your being.

2. On an in-breath, bend your right leg, bring it towards your pelvis and place it on the outside of your left leg, foot flat on the floor as close to the left hip as is comfortable.

3. Bend your left knee, keeping your left upper thigh flat on the floor. Now draw in your left leg so that your left foot comes to rest beside your right glute. Your hips remain square and forwards, bottom seated on the ground.

4. Lengthen your spine skywards, pulling up your lower abdominals. On an in-breath, raise your right arm skywards, then lower it to a resting position on the floor behind the centre of your back. At the same time, gently twist your upper torso from your hip in the direction of your right hand.

5. On an in-breath, raise your left arm skywards, then either bring this arm to wrap around your right thigh hugging it towards your torso, or you can hook the left elbow outside of the right knee, with lower arm and hand pointing skywards.

6. Take a few breaths here, breathing in to elongate the spine upwards and open the chest area. You may also choose to gently increase the twist on each out-breath.

7. To come out of the pose, release your arms, gently bring your upper torso to face forwards again and place both hands flat on the floor to the outside of your right foot to counteract the twist. Take a few breaths, then return to Step 1.

8. Repeat the above sequence, but twist in the opposite direction, starting with the left leg.

Tip:
*   Place a yoga block under your downward hand to help keep the body aligned.

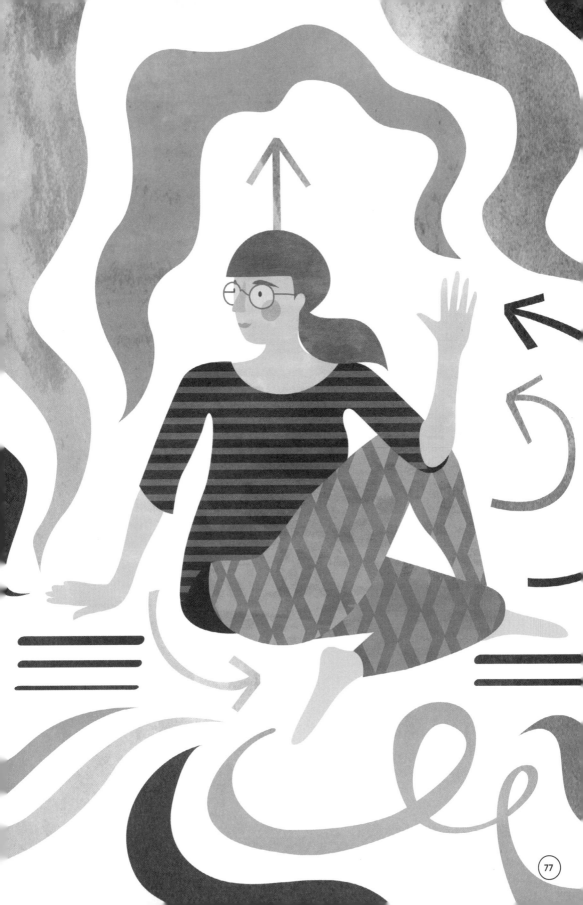

SPHINX

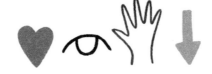

Salamba bhujangasana

A sphinx is a mythological creature with the head of a human, the body of a lion and the wings of a falcon. The famous Great Sphinx of Giza, the huge limestone statue guarding the Egyptian pyramids by the Nile, provides a good visual reference for this bold stance. In yoga, Sphinx pose is a gentle backbend, which opens the lungs and the heart centre of the chest and strengthens the lower back. It also activates and tones the core, glutes and leg muscles, calms the mind and provides space to connect with your inner strength.

Here's how to explore the pose:

1. Begin by lying flat on your front, legs outstretched behind you, hip-width apart. The tops of your feet press into the mat as your toes spread and extend away from your body. Forehead rests on the mat.

2. Stretch your arms along the floor out in front of you, keeping them flat on the mat and parallel to each other, fingers gently splayed and your middle finger pointing forwards.

3. On an in-breath, raise your head and chest off the ground, then slide your arms back towards your body until the elbows are directly beneath the shoulders. Roll your shoulder blades down and back, opening your chest to the front and extending your neck and head skywards. Keep the face soft and looking forwards.

4. Keeping your stomach and hips flat on your mat, engage your core muscles and press downwards through your pubic region. Lengthen your tailbone downwards and backwards towards your legs and toes. Activate your glutes and the muscles in your legs, turning your thighs inwards and gently engaging your kneecaps.

5. Breathe here. Relax your face and, if you wish to, close your eyes. If your eyes are closed, direct your gaze to the centre of your forehead to connect more fully to the peace within.

6. To come out of the pose, on an out-breath, lower your head and chest to the mat, bring your arms to rest alongside your body (palms upwards), turn your head to one side and take a few restful breaths.

7. When ready, come to kneeling and then fold forwards to relax in Child's pose (page 108).

Tip:
* If you would like to reduce the intensity of the backbend here, gently ease your elbows further out in front of you.

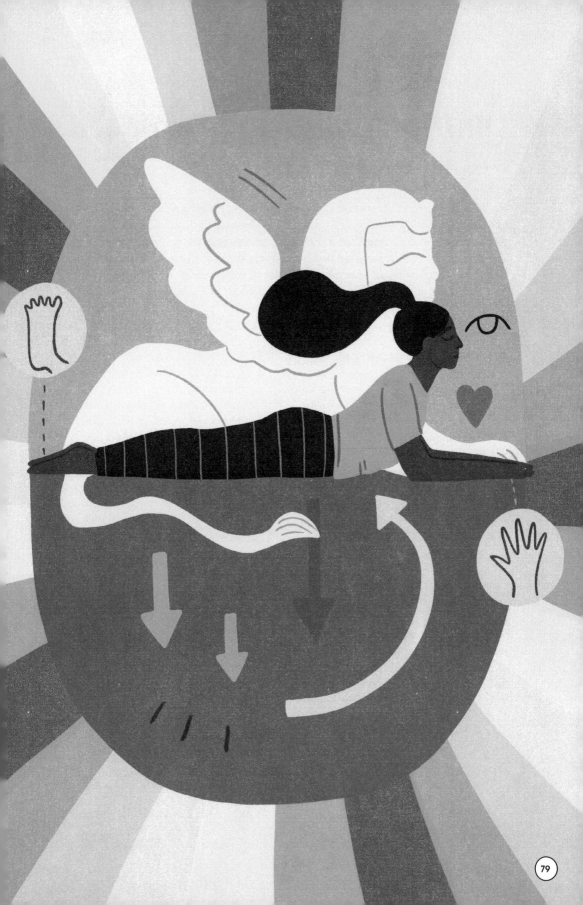

UPWARD-FACING DOG

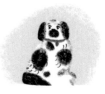

Urdhva mukha svanasana

As befits its canine reference, Upward-facing dog works on the energies of the heart. An advanced pose, it opens the chest area, releases tension in the neck and shoulders, lengthens the spine and strengthens the muscles in the arms and legs. It can also be therapeutic for asthma, stimulate digestion and support the flow of energy within the body, helping to lift fatigue and low mood. Anyone who has carpal tunnel syndrome or experiences back or wrist injuries should not practise this pose.

Here's how to explore the pose:

1. Lie flat on your stomach, legs in line with your hips, with your tailbone pointing towards your heels and the tops of your feet pressing into the floor. Your forehead is resting gently on the mat.

2. Bend your elbows, then bring your hands to lie flat on the ground next to your ribcage, with your fingers spread and pointing forwards. Tuck your elbows right in to your ribs, your legs are flat on the ground, in line with your hips.

3. Using the muscles in your legs and calves, lift your kneecaps. Engage your core by drawing your navel towards your spine, extending your neck forwards.

4. On an in-breath, press into your hands and feet, push your chest forwards through the arms and roll your shoulder blades back and down. Lift your chest and legs off the floor, so the full weight of your body is supported by your hands and feet.

5. You can direct your gaze forwards or upwards, whichever feels most comfortable, but aim to elongate your neck rather than crunching it into the spine. If at any point you feel a pinching or pain in your back, release back down and rest in Child's pose (page 108). To do this, sit back on your heels with knees hip-width apart, before lowering your torso towards your thighs and gently placing the forehead on the floor in front of you. Your arms can be stretched out in front or parallel with the thighs behind.

6. If you feel at ease in Upward-facing dog, take a few comfortable breaths, before gently lowering yourself and pushing back to rest in Child's pose (as described above).

Tip:

* Some practitioners might find it helpful to become comfortable with Cobra pose (page 86) ahead of practising Upward-facing dog.

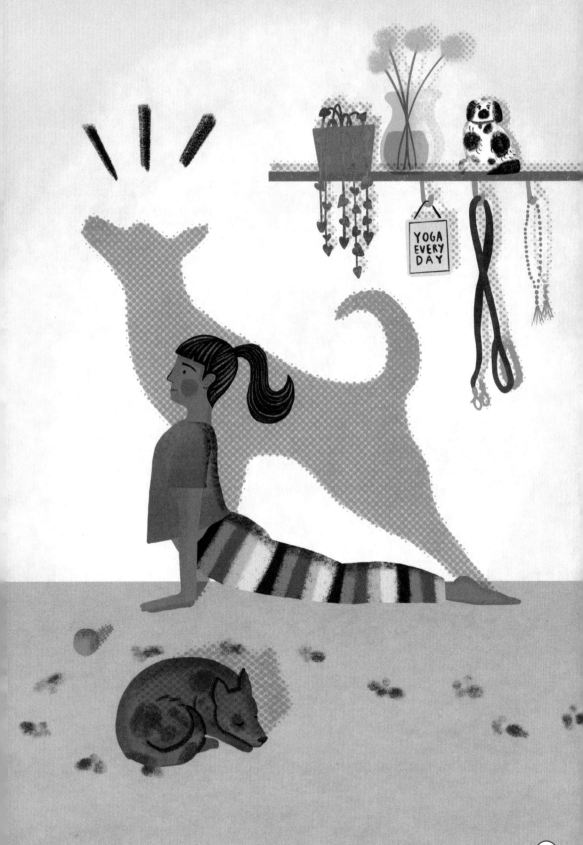

LIZARD

Utthan pristhasana

Lizards are animals of resilience and innovation, able to survive in the harshest terrain, regenerate body parts and camouflage to blend in with surroundings. You can breathe new life into your mind and body with Lizard pose, which stretches your hamstrings, hip flexors and quadriceps. This is an advanced posture, so it's important to listen to your body and ease into it gently. Before beginning, warm up with a round of Sun salutations (page 116).

Here's how to explore the pose:

1. Begin on all fours in tabletop position (Step 2, page 62) and then flow into Downward-facing dog (page 72).

2. On an out-breath, step your right foot forwards to the outside of your right hand, bringing your toes in line with your fingers. Your knee is bent at a right angle above your ankles, forming a lunge position. To assist balance, turn your right foot slightly outwards, 45 degrees, and direct the centre of your knee in the same direction as your middle toe.

3. Lower your left knee to the ground, press into your hip, while keeping your arms and back straight, drawing your chestbone away from your waist and keeping your head forwards and in line with your spine.

4. On an in-breath, bring your elbows to the floor beneath your shoulders, with your forearms flat on the ground in front of them, palms flat on the ground. If this is uncomfortable or difficult, place your forearms on a block. If this still feels too intense – or is painful – try staying on your palms and keep your arms straight.

5. Press up onto the ball of your left foot as you straighten your left leg. Again, if this feels too much, keep your knee on the ground and gradually build up to this position with practice over time.

6. Take a few comfortable breaths in the pose and, when ready, gently release. On an out-breath, straighten your arms and bring your wrists to below your shoulders. Then, on an in-breath, step back into Downward-facing dog and breathe steadily as you prepare to repeat Lizard on the other side of your body.

7. Step forwards with your left foot to repeat the sequence.

8. Once completed, slowly come down and rest in Child's pose (page 108).

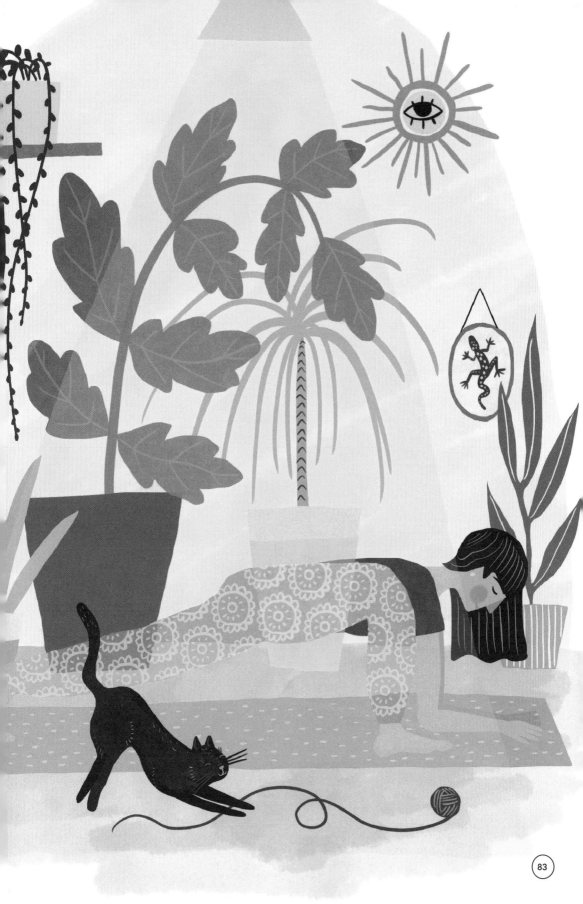

DOLPHIN

Ardha pincha mayurasana

Sociable and playful, dolphins can send and hear sonic frequencies that are 10 times the upper limit of adult humans, travel through water at speeds of 55km per hour, and they display compassion, rescuing other animals and even people. As a pose, Dolphin builds strength in the upper body, especially the arms, shoulders and back. Anyone who has shoulder, neck, head or eye injuries or suffers from high blood pressure should not practise this pose.

Here's how to explore the pose:

1. Warm up your shoulders by shrugging them up and down and rotating them backwards and forwards. Then warm up the wrists by clasping your hands together and rotating them gently.

2. Begin by positioning yourself on all fours in tabletop (Step 2, page 62). Pay close attention to the alignment of your shoulders, arms and wrists and ensure your legs are extending straight out directly behind your knees. Take a few breaths to calm, focus and ground yourself.

3. Lower your elbows to the floor, so they are directly below your shoulder sockets. Place your lower arms flat on the floor directly in front of your elbows with your palms facing downwards, fingers slightly splayed like a dolphin's fin.

4. On an in-breath, turn your toes under, pull your shoulder blades back and open your chest. Keep your lower arms flat on the floor.

5. On the same in-breath, pushing through your arms, upper body and legs, raise your hips skywards so your back legs are straight (without locking the knees) and there's another straight line from your hips down towards your head. Let the neck and head hang freely. The forehead can rest softly on your mat. Lower the heels towards the floor as far as is comfortable.

6. Take a few deep breaths and imagine you're a graceful dolphin surfing the waves. Then gently bend the knees, untuck the toes, lower the hips and return to tabletop.

7. When you're ready, slowly walk your hands back and bring your body up to kneeling, with your head coming up last. Gently roll out your wrists to release any tension and take a few deep breaths.

Tips:
* As with Downward-facing dog (page 72), you may find it easier to have your knees slightly bent at Step 5, and only stretch the heels to a point that feels comfortable.
* Another option at Step 5 is to clasp your hands together so that they form a tripod shape with your lower arms.

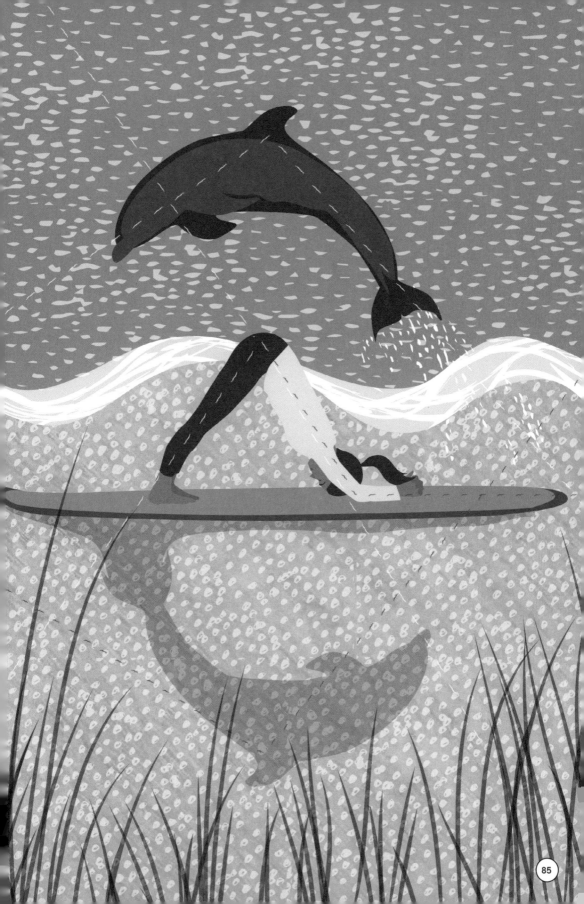

COBRA

Bhujangasana

A powerful pose, Cobra strengthens the spine, gluteal muscles, thighs, arms and shoulders. It also helps to open the chest and encourages the release of tension in the shoulders and neck.

Here's how to explore the pose:

1. Lie face down, legs together, tops of your feet resting on the floor, soles facing skywards, forehead gently placed on your mat. Place your palms flat on the floor, underneath your shoulders, keeping your fingers pointing forwards and your elbows close to your body.

2. Take a moment here, gently breathing in and out through the nose. Tune into your being and imagine what it might be like to be a cobra slithering along the earth. Lengthen your spine and crown of your head forwards, while pressing your pelvis and legs earthwards.

3. To raise your cobra skywards, on an in-breath, engage your core stomach muscles to lift your upper torso forwards and upwards to a position that does not strain your back. Only come up as far as feels comfortable and keep pressing into the earth with your legs and pelvis.

4. Open your chest and broaden your collarbone, lifting and rolling your shoulders back and down. Keep your elbows slightly bent, hands supporting you on the ground. Feel the lovely elongation of the spine and opening of the chest area. Continue to press down with your lower body.

5. Take a few breaths here, then slowly sink back down to the ground. Observe the different sensations that flow through your being when you're an earthbound cobra and facing skywards.

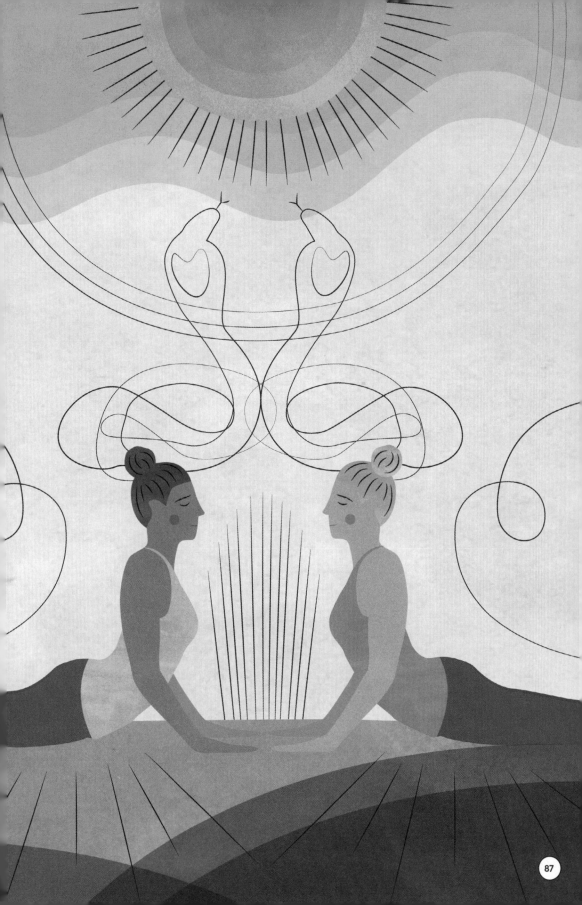

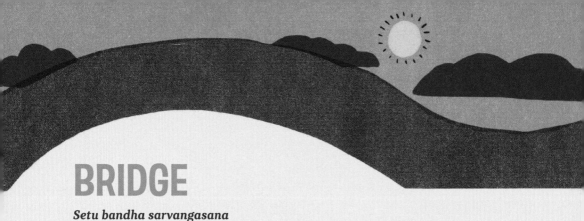

BRIDGE

Setu bandha sarvangasana

All over the world, bridges are used to provide a link between one location and another. In yoga, Bridge pose is said to assist with building a connection with the higher self. The heart is the way, the bridge between worlds. This gentle inversion, meaning the heart is higher from the ground than the head, stimulates the abdominal organs and thyroid gland, while stretching the spine, hip flexors and thighs.

Here's how to explore the pose:

1. Lie flat on your back, legs outstretched and in line with the hips, arms alongside your body, palms down and resting on the ground. Take a few breaths here.

2. On an in-breath, bend your knees, and draw your feet towards – but not touching – your buttocks. Keep your feet and knees hip-distance apart. Exhale.

3. On another in-breath, press down evenly through your feet and lift your hips off the floor. If this is difficult, you may find it helpful to place a yoga block or a bolster under your sacrum (the triangular bone at the bottom of your spine). Exhale.

4. Again, on an in-breath, open your shoulders, drawing your shoulder blades towards each other. From here, press down through the shoulders into the ground and lift your chest skywards, raising your lower back and bottom off the floor.

5. Bring your hands together beneath your sacrum and link your fingers while extending your arms towards your feet. If this feels too much, keep the arms flat (palms down) alongside your body. Keep your neck and head flat on the mat with your gaze directed upwards. Take a few comfortable breaths.

6. When ready, unclasp your hands and move your arms back to alongside your body. Release your shoulders and slowly lower your spine, beginning from your shoulders and, vertebrae by vertebrae, working your way to your buttocks, until your back is flat on the ground.

7. Take a few breaths, then bend your knees, bring them to your chest, give them a hug and gently rock back and forth or from side to side to counteract the Bridge pose. When ready, release your legs and extend them flat along your mat.

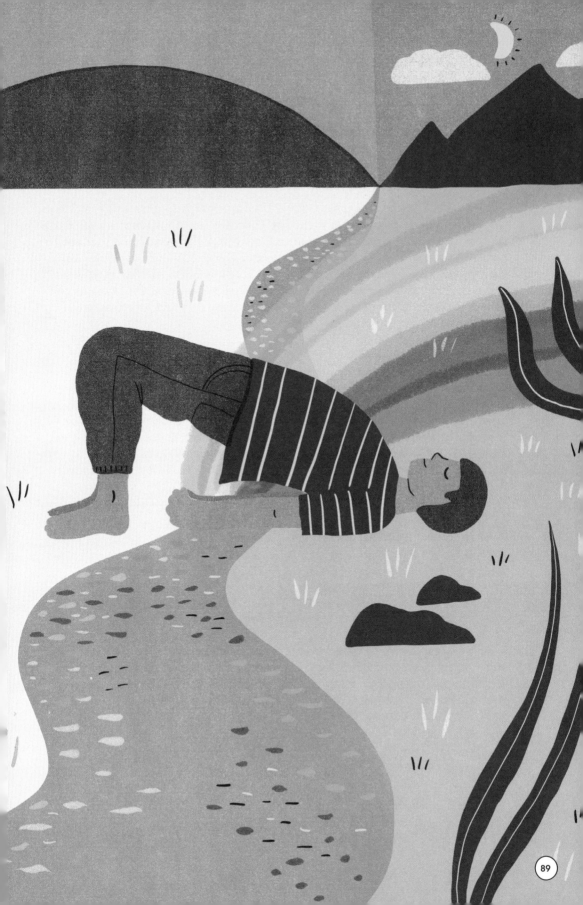

LOCUST

Salabhasana

The locust is a fascinating insect. Mostly, it's a solitary creature, but sometimes they come together and become a powerful unit. They're a dramatic reminder of what can be achieved when communities and individuals unite and take action. Locust pose is a dynamic backbend that strengthens the back, buttocks and legs. It also stretches the spine, opens the chest and heart, and stimulates the stomach region. Make sure to warm up fully and be gentle on your back as you ease into the pose. Progress slowly as you continue through your practice.

Here's how to explore the pose:

1. Begin by lying flat on your stomach (you might wish to place a folded blanket under the hips for comfort) with your forehead gently resting on the ground. Your arms are alongside your body (palms upwards) and your legs stretch out behind you (soles of the feet face upwards). Take a few breaths to calm and centre your being.

2. Shifting the weight of your torso forwards, roll your shoulder blades up and back, lift your head (keep the gaze towards the ground) and open up your chest area. Extend your legs backwards through the soles of your feet. Keep your hips, stomach, arms and legs pressed towards the ground.

3. On an in-breath, engage the muscles in your legs and buttocks. Extend the legs backwards, raising them off the ground to a comfortable height, while continuing to extend backwards and upwards through your feet.

4. When ready, lift your extended arms (palms up) to a comfortable height off the ground, extending the fingertips towards the feet. The shoulder blades are lifted and rolled back, as if you're unfurling and opening wings backwards, with your chest opening away from the ground.

5. Keep your gaze forwards, with your chin lowered and the back of your neck long and relaxed.

6. Take a few comfortable breaths here, then lower back to the ground, lay your head to one side and breathe for a moment. You may wish to repeat the sequence a second time and turn the head to the opposite side at the end of the pose. When ready, come to all fours in tabletop (Step 2, page 62) and then sit back into Child's pose (page 108).

BOW

Dhanurasana

The moment you start pulling back on a bowstring, potential energy is stored in the flexing limb, ready to send the arrow soaring. Similarly, Bow pose activates the energy centres of the heart and core areas of the body. A strong backbend, it stretches the hip flexors and hamstrings as well as the muscles in the back, chest and neck. It can help with fatigue and digestion, while also easing tension in the lower back caused by sitting for long periods. Before beginning, warm up your body with a round of Sun salutations (page 116).

Here's how to explore the pose:

1. Begin by lying on your front, arms resting alongside your body with palms facing upwards. Your legs are hip-width apart, with the tops of the feet resting on the mat and toes pointing away from the body. Forehead gently rests on the mat.

2. On an out-breath, bend your knees and bring your heels close to your buttocks, keeping the toes pointed.

3. Lift your arms up and gently reach back to take hold of your ankles from the outside. If you can't quite make it, place a yoga strap around your ankles to extend your reach, but still be careful not to overstretch or twist the body.

4. On an in-breath, press down through your pubic region, draw your lower belly in and up, and lift and roll your shoulder blades back towards each other. At the same time, lengthen your spine forwards and upwards, opening the chest area. Extend your neck upwards, keeping your head facing forwards.

5. Engage the muscles in your legs and, on an in-breath, press your ankles into your hands, lifting your chest and thighs off the ground. Keep the knees hip-distance apart.

6. Take a few comfortable breaths here, then gently release to lie flat on the ground. Breathe, then come to a kneeling position before folding forwards into Child's pose (page 108).

Tip:

* Be gentle on yourself in Bow pose. This is an intermediate pose and many practitioners find it challenging. Never overstretch to the point of pain.

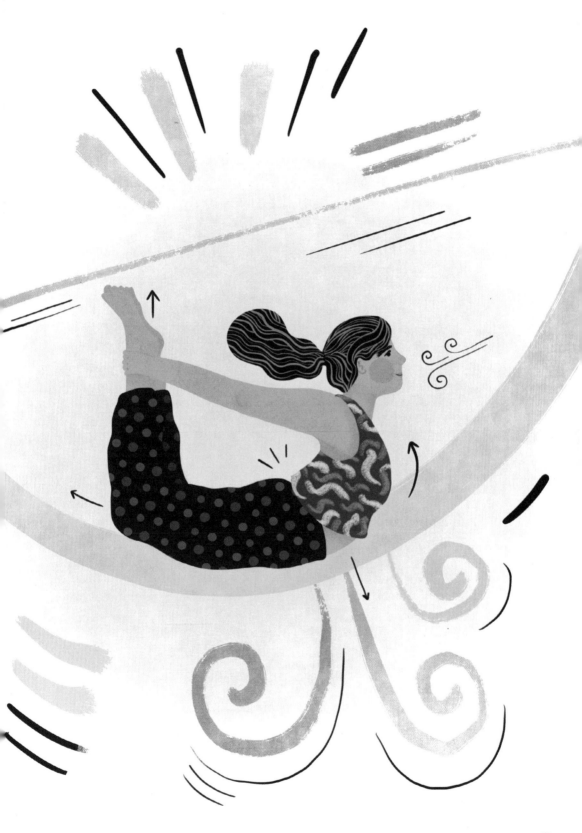

CAMEL

Ustrasana

The word camel comes from the Arabic *jamal*, which conveys the idea of beauty. Camel is a strong pose that works on the energy centres around the heart, supporting the blossom of love and compassion. It also builds strength and flexibility in the back and opens the chest and throat. In advance of your practice, it's wise to fully warm up the spine with a round of Sun salutations (page 116), then ease yourself into the pose gently. Anyone who has any back, neck, head or heart conditions is advised not to practise Camel pose.

Here's how to explore the pose:

1. Come to upright kneeling on your mat. You may wish to place a folded blanket under your knees for extra cushioning. Your knees are hip-width apart, with your shins and the tops of your feet pressing downwards. The hands are in Prayer pose (Step 6, page 21). Take a few breaths and connect with your core.

2. On an in-breath, take your hands to rest on your lower back, palms on the top of your bottom with the fingers flowing down, thumbs facing upwards (see top inset, opposite). On another in-breath, lengthen down through your spine and tuck your tailbone forwards, keeping thighs and hips at an angle of 90 degrees to the floor. Engage your inner thighs by pressing them towards each other.

3. Again, on an in-breath, draw your spine upwards, lift and roll the shoulders back – drawing the shoulder blades towards each other at the back – and gently flow your upper chest to opening skywards. The shoulders slowly move back and down.

4. Gently reach down with the right hand and place it on the right heel, then place the left hand on the left heel. If this feels too much or causes pain, tuck your toes under, bringing your feet at right angles to the floor (see bottom inset, opposite), and within easier reach. If you feel discomfort, slowly return to the upright kneeling pose.

5. Take a few comfortable breaths. To come out of the pose, tuck in the chin and bring your hands back to your lower back as before. On an in-breath, bring yourself up, starting from the base of your spine and slowly drawing up your chest to face the front. The neck and head come up last.

6. Release your hands from the lower back, sit gently on your heels and flow forwards to rest for a few moments in Child's pose (page 108).

Tips:

* Some practitioners find it helpful to place yoga blocks at the outside of each foot at the beginning of the pose and then rest their hands on them at Step 4.

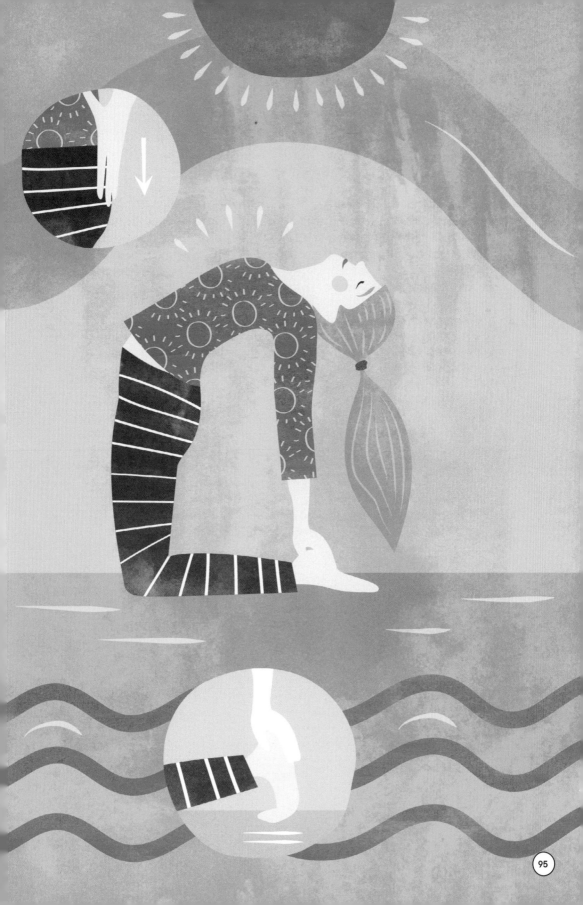

CONQUEROR'S BREATH

Ujjayi pranayama

Awareness and control of the breath is central to yoga (page 16) and there are many techniques that help to build a greater understanding of how to channel its strengths in everyday life as well as your practice. Conqueror's, or Ocean's, breath aids focus and improves positivity. It can also help to generate internal heat, ease respiratory problems and reduce stress and anxiety.

Here's how to explore the technique:

1. Sit comfortably on your yoga mat, tall and upright, straight spine, relaxed shoulders and face. Your eyes can be open or closed, whichever you find most comfortable.

2. Sit for a moment, breathing at your regular pace, and allow your body and mind to relax.

3. Take a deep breath in through both nostrils and bring the breath up into the top of the throat. As you begin to exhale, open your mouth to create a round shape and flow the breath out through the mouth – just as you would breathe when fogging up a mirror, making a strong 'HA' sound.

4. Practise this breathflow for a couple of minutes and focus on feeling how the air travels through the throat and out through the mouth.

5. When comfortable with this breathflow, you're ready to move on to Conqueror's breath. Close your mouth and repeat the breathflow described above, but when you come to exhale, do so through the nose. On the out-breath, you will observe a gentle ocean sound as the breath flows up along the curved back of the throat.

6. Try to keep the breathing ratio steady, so the exhalation is twice the length of the inhalation (1:2).

Tips:

* For beginners, it's sensible to limit your practice of Conqueror's breath – in through the nose and out through the nose – to no longer than five minutes. Observe how your mind and body feels afterwards. (Longer lengths of time can be practised when you've gained more experience of this breathwork.)

* Whenever you find yourself in a situation where you're feeling anxious and stressed, think – and practise – Conqueror's breath to help you regain control.

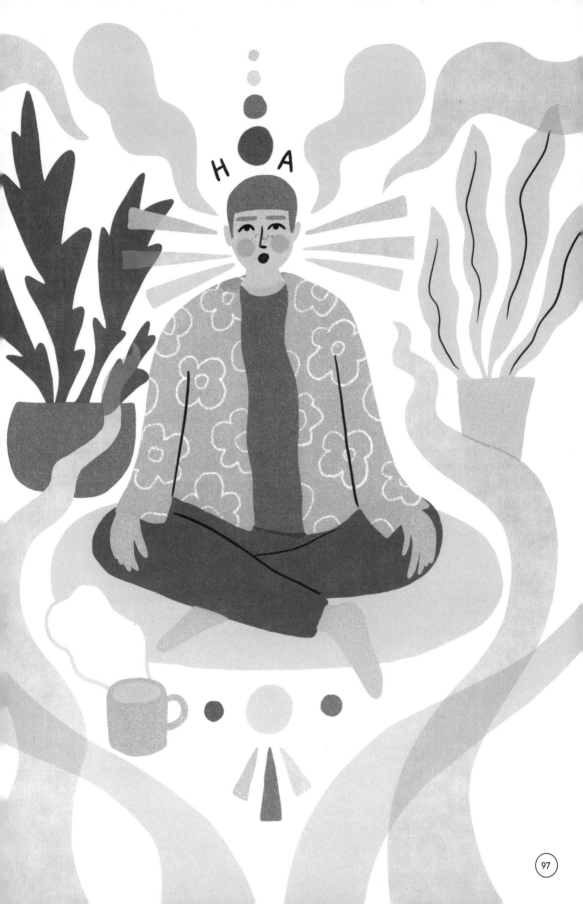

LION'S BREATH

Simhasana pranayama

The lion has been a symbol of strength, courage, honour, nobility and pride since ancient times, with a roar that can be heard up to 8km away. So, it's no surprise that Lion's breath is a powerful breathing exercise, which boosts strength, vitality and confidence, while supporting self-expression.

Here's how to explore the technique:

1. Take up a kneeling position on your mat, back straight and upright, shoulders opening backwards and coming down, palms resting on thighs (above the knee), fingers spread like lion claws.

2. Breathe in through both nostrils – imagine the breath reaching all the way up to the crown of your head. As you do this, maintain a straight spine, keep the shoulders pulled back and down, and the chest wide.

3. As you breathe out, gently lean your body forwards, open your mouth wide, stick your tongue out long and flat pointing downwards towards the ground, and make a strong 'HA' sound. At the same time, bring your gaze skywards, up through the middle of your eyes.

4. When the breath is expelled, draw your tongue back in, close your mouth, bring your eyes back to looking forwards and straighten your spine into a strong upright position, remembering to check that your shoulders are coming down, away from your ears.

5. Repeat this breathflow for about five or 10 breaths and observe how you feel.

6. Try varying your Lion's breath. From your upright kneeling position, take your knees wide with your palms on the floor (wrists turned so that your fingers are pointing towards your body – see image, opposite). Breathe in through your nostrils as you tilt your upper body forwards (push downwards through your arms and maintain a straight spine). As before, on an out-breath, stick your tongue out long and flat pointing downwards, while your gaze moves skywards through the middle of your eyes.

Tip:

* Have a play with this breath and your body. Channel the inner strength of a lion as you practise different stretches.

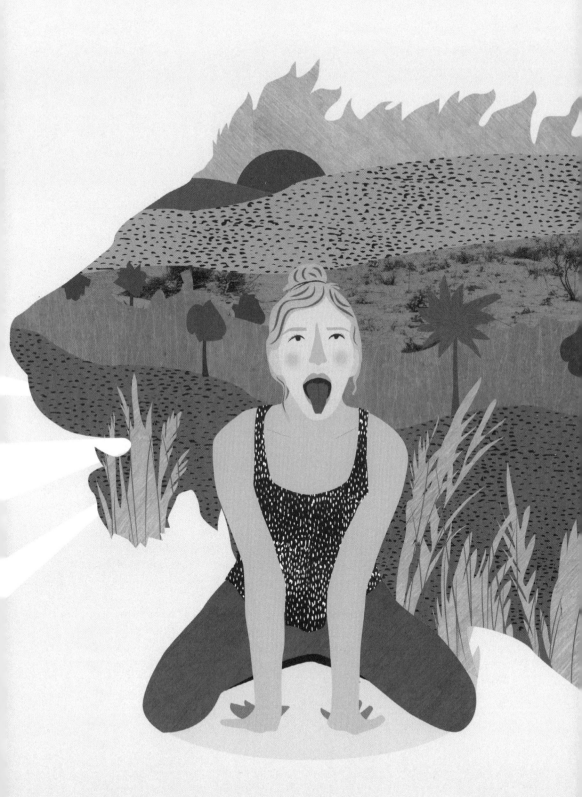

BUMBLEBEE BREATH

Bhramari pranayama

Bees are amazing creatures. The head on a honeybee has 170 odour receptors, making its sense of smell precise enough to tell whether a plant contains pollen or nectar from miles away and detect the difference between hundreds of flowers. Their famous buzzing noise is the sound of their wings thrumming at speeds of up to 200 times per second as they bumble along. Bumblebee breath aims to imitate their steady humming sound. This method calms the mind, reduces anxiety and soothes the airways and throat. It's also thought to help with digestion.

Here's how to explore the technique:

1. Sit in a comfortable position with your spine tall, crown of the head extended, face soft, shoulders relaxed and away from your ears. You could be cross-legged on your mat or sitting upright in a chair with a solid back.

2. You may choose to have your eyes open or closed, whichever feels most comfortable. Closing them helps to reduce distractions from outside. It also directs your attention inwards so you can focus on what's happening there.

3. Take your hands towards the sides of your head, place your index fingers on the tragus (the bit between your cheek and ear) and gently press to close the entrance to the ear canal.

4. Take a deep breath in through both nostrils. Then breathe out slowly through the mouth, making a humming or buzzing sound in the back of your throat. Your lips should be lightly touching, with your upper and lower teeth slightly separated.

5. Make the buzzing sound as you exhale for whatever length of time feels comfortable. Observe the vibrations of the buzzing in your head and throat. You can explore the sensation of different buzzing tones.

6. Repeat six or seven times or for a period that feels right for you. When you've finished your practice, remain seated quietly and enjoy the moment.

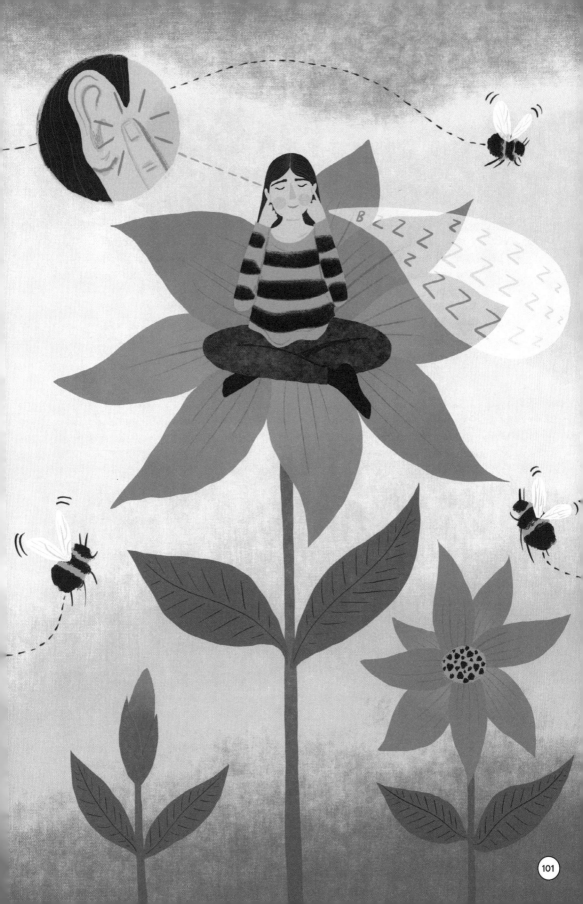

BREATHE INTO BRAVERY

Want to find your inner strength, but also calm your nerves? You might like to try the following exercise. To be brave is to show mental or moral strength in the face of danger, fear or difficulty. It feels safe and easy to stay within your comfort zone, but personal growth comes from going beyond it from time to time. Stepping outside its boundaries allows you to take on new challenges, boost your skills and expand the size of your comfort zone. So, how can you harness this strength when feeling anxious? There are many different methods available, but here's one breathing exercise that uses the power of self-love to overcome fear.

Here's how to explore the technique:

1. Start the exercise in a comfortable seated position of your choice, either on your mat or in a chair. Hold your posture tall and upright, head facing forwards, chest open, shoulders back and down.

2. To enhance the flow of energy physically, consciously and subconsciously, position your hands in *Ganesh mudra*. To do this, bring your elbows up to heart level, place your left hand in front of your heart (turned sideways, palm facing away from you, thumb pointing downwards and fingers bent). Then bring your right palm across your chest and hook the fingers of both hands together (elbows aligned horizontally and pointing out, see right).

3. Along with *Ganesh mudra*, the words 'I am' will be used. These two words are often used to affirm positive qualities. Here, the affirmation is: 'I am brave.'

4. Seated comfortably – and with your hands forming *Ganesh mudra* – take a deep breath in through both nostrils. As you breathe in for a count of three, say one word in your mind on each count:

* I
* Am
* Brave

Hold the breath for a count of two. Exhale slowly through the nostrils for a count of six, repeating 'I am brave' twice along to your six counts:

* I
* Am
* Brave
* I
* Am
* Brave

5. On the extended out-breath, pull the elbows away from each other, keeping the fingers locked together. Feel the muscles in your arms, chest and heart activate, as well as an increased flow of heart energy.

6. Relax. Repeat the breathwork for eight rounds. After you're done, sit for a moment and observe any sensations.

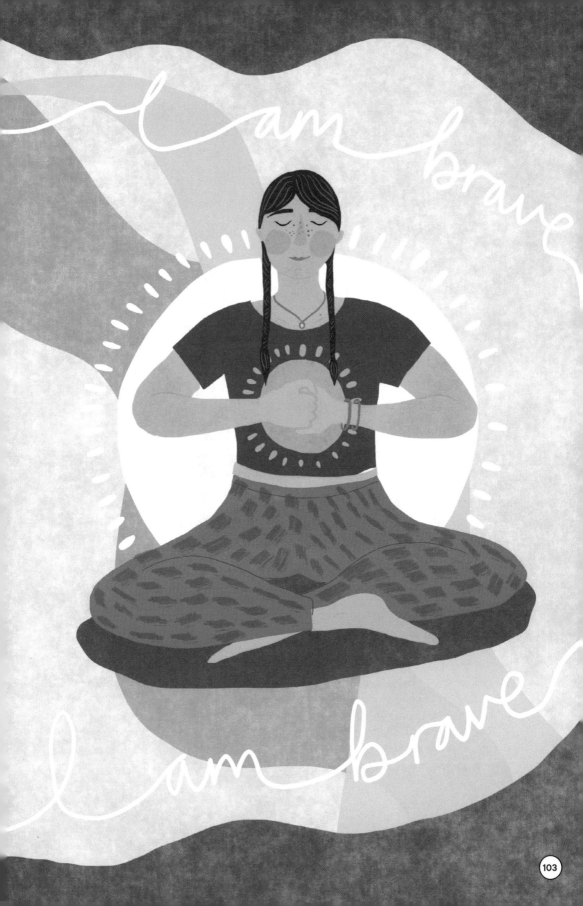

BOX BREATHING

Sama vritti pranayama

The square is a sacred geometric shape in which all sides are equal. In yoga, Box breathing is a technique that harnesses this equality for the rhythm and flow of the breath, helping to bring mind and body into harmony, and lowering the stress hormone, cortisol, and blood pressure. It's a great way to ease feelings of stress or anxiety, as it helps to calm the mind, enabling you to think around problems more clearly.

Here's how to explore the technique:

1. Sit in a comfortable position. You can, however, practise this technique lying down or even standing up if needed. You may choose to follow Conqueror's breath (page 96), by breathing in and out through the nose. You can also opt to have your eyes open or closed, whichever feels most comfortable. Closing them helps to draw the focus inwards.

2. Take a deep breath, then follow this four-step pattern. The pace of the count isn't so important, but try to remember to keep all the counts equal, just as the sides of a box measure the same length:
    * Breathe in for a count of four.
    * Hold the breath for a count of four.
    * Breathe out for a count of four.
    * Hold for a count of four.

3. Repeat this four-step pattern for a few minutes or as long as feels comfortable. Observe the effects on your being.

4. At first, it may be difficult to keep the count of four, so you could start with with a lower figure, say two, for example:
    * Breathe in for a count of two.
    * Hold the breath for a count of two.
    * Breathe out for a count of two.
    * Hold for a count of two.
From here, you can gradually work your way up to a count of four.

5. You can use this exercise, as well as Breathe into bravery (page 102) and Cooling breath (page 106), whenever you'd like to bring calm to your inner being.

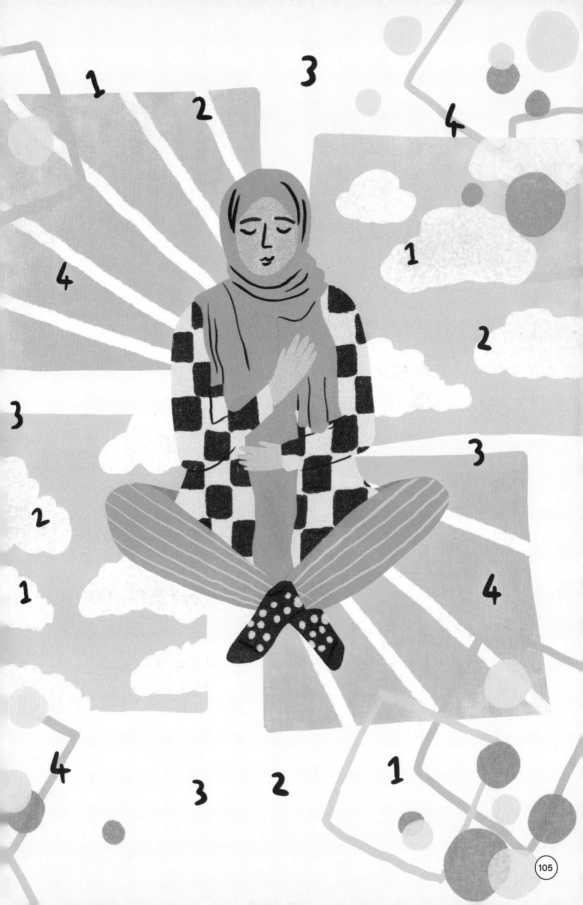

COOLING BREATH

Sitali pranayama

Whether it's a hot summer's afternoon or you've been cooped up indoors in a stuffy room all day with the rain lashing down outside, this breathing exercise – done with a rolled tongue – will lower the body heat and calm the mind.

Here's how to explore the technique:

1. Start in a comfortable seated position of your choice, either on your mat or in a chair. Keep your spine upright and straight, shoulders relaxed and open.

2. Gently rest your hands on your knees, palms open and facing upwards or fingers held in a *mudra* position. You could try *Gyan mudra* (Step 4, page 44). This is said to activate the area in the brain related to wisdom and knowledge.

3. Sit for a moment, breathing in your normal pattern, to allow your body to settle and your senses to relax and centre.

4. Breathing in through the nose, form a circular 'O' with your lips. Curl your tongue, bringing up the sides to form a 'U' shape. Gently push your tongue through the open circle your mouth has made so that it comfortably extends beyond the lips.

5. Take a deep breath in through the mouth along the straw-like tongue, then slowly draw your tongue back into the mouth, close the lips, hold the breath and breathe out through your nose. Repeat this technique to a simple rhythm, breathing in for a count of five, holding for a count of two and exhaling for a count of five.

6. If you are unable to curl your tongue, there is an alternative cooling technique called *Sitkari pranayama*. Bring your teeth together (mouth open) and inhale through the gaps in your closed teeth. Close your lips, hold the breath and breathe out through your nose, following the same count as Step 5.

7. Whichever cooling breathing technique you practise, continue for two to three minutes. Relax and return to your regular breathing pattern.

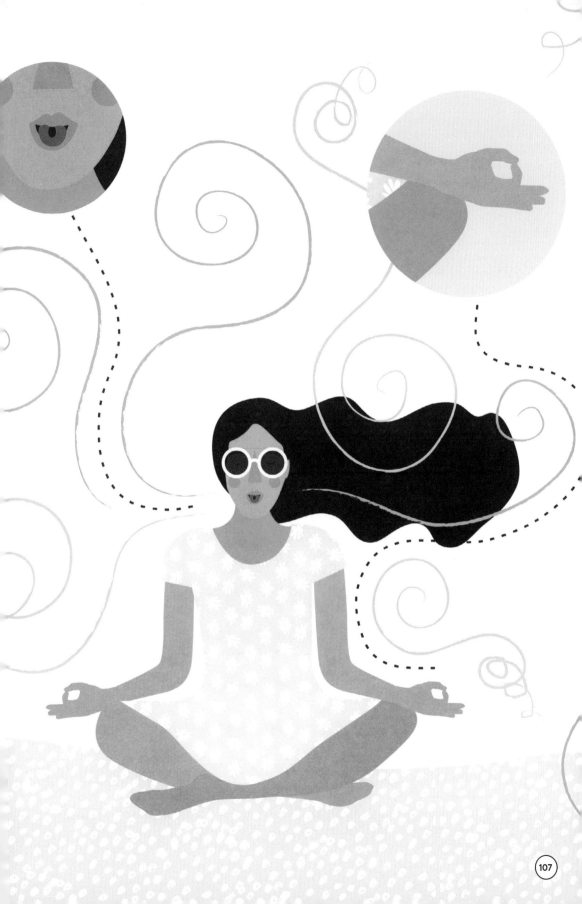

CHILD'S POSE

Balasana

A lovely, nurturing yoga position, Child's pose resembles a baby curled up in the womb. It can be practised any time – either by itself or between other poses – to calm and soothe the brain and help the body to release stress and return to a place of balance, security and composure.

Here's how to explore the pose:

1. Start in a kneeling position on your mat, your bottom towards or resting on your heels. The knees can be together or open, hip-width apart, with your big toes touching at the back. Your arms are loose by your sides, palms facing the body.

2. Take a few deep breaths. On an in-breath, lift your arms skywards, stretching them straight up either side of your head (palms facing each other).

3. On an out-breath, lower your upper torso so that it folds forwards over your thighs or, if your thighs are apart, between them. Bring your forehead to rest gently on your mat with your arms flowing and stretching backwards along the outside of your legs, palms facing upwards.

4. Rest here. Allow your body to surrender in this position. Spread and push back, lengthening your spine, while opening and releasing your shoulders (your forehead remains on the mat).

5. Relax in this position for a few minutes. Breathe deeply and observe its calming effect on your mind and body.

6. When you're ready to come out of the pose, bring your hands forwards (palms facing downwards) to either side of your knees and, breathing in, raise your torso back to your kneeling position at Step 1.

7. Take a few deep breaths and be reminded of the benefits of nurturing body, mind and spirit.

....

Tips:

✳ Some practitioners like to rest their forehead on a folded blanket, while others find it more comfortable to raise the floor to them by resting their forehead on a yoga block or their crossed hands.

✳ If it feels uncomfortable keeping the arms behind, stretch them out in front of you, shoulder-width apart, palms touching the floor.

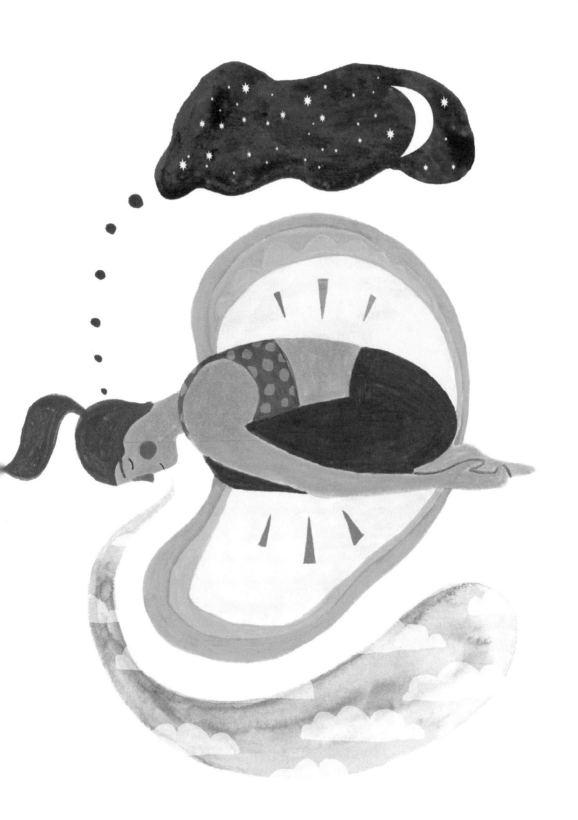

EXTENDED PUPPY POSE

Uttana shishosana

The unconditional love of these bouncing bundles of canine joy is reflected in Extended puppy pose, which warms body and mind. It also releases tension in the arms, shoulders, neck and upper and lower back, while helping to relieve stress and build self-confidence.

Here's how to explore the pose:

1. Begin on all fours in tabletop position (Step 2, page 62) on a soft, non-slip surface.

2. From here, walk your hands in front of you to a comfortable stretched position. On an in-breath, extend your spine forwards reaching through your arms and fingers. Allow your forehead to rest gently on the floor (you may wish to use a folded blanket here). Your shoulders and chest stay off the ground – at a level lower than your bottom – opening and releasing downwards. If it helps, bend the elbows and have the lower arms resting on the ground, palms flat and fingers extending forwards.

3. Simultaneously extend your spine forwards through your arms and backwards through your sacrum, lifting your tailbone skywards.

4. Take a moment to breathe and explore this stretch. Think about the movement and how your muscles feel.

5. When ready, slowly walk the hands back towards your body, returning the torso to either upright kneeling or with your bottom touching your heels, whichever is most comfortable. The head comes up last. Take a few breaths and, if you wish, gently flex your wrists to release any tension.

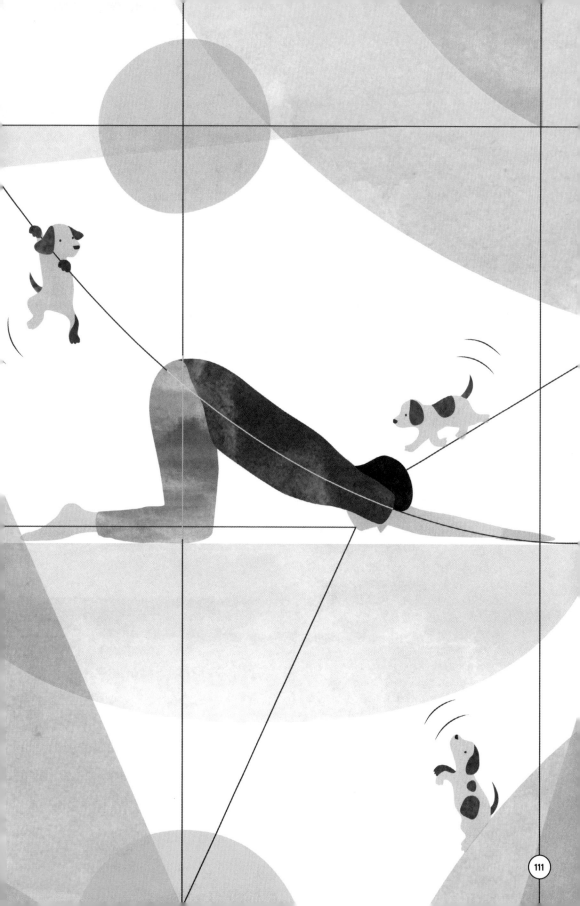

LEGS UP THE WALL

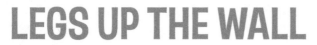

Viparita karani

The modern world is fast-paced, with lots to do every day. But it's important to make sure a busy schedule has a few free periods when you can rest and enjoy some downtime. A gentle inversion that's just the trick is Legs up the wall. Often practised towards the end of a yoga class, it relaxes the mind, calms the nervous system, supports the flow of blood back to the body, helps to ease anxiety and stress, and reduces tension in the legs. Overall, it's a great stress-relieving pose that can be done whenever you feel the need to relax, restore and reconnect with yourself.

Here's how to explore the pose:

1. Sit straight and tall close to a wall, legs slightly to one side and your bottom near the wall but not touching it. You might like to have a soft blanket on top of your yoga mat for added cushioning.

2. Gently lower your back to lying flat on the floor, then slowly swing your legs up the wall so they are softly resting against it. Your arms can fall loosely at the side of your body, palms gradually opening upwards.

3. Stay lying down, with your legs resting up against the wall, gently breathing in and out. You can keep your eyes open or closed, whichever feels right for you. If you choose to keep them open, try to keep the gaze soft and fixed on one point to avoid distractions.

4. Stay in the position for as long as you find helpful and is comfortable. If your room's a little chilly, you might find it nice to cover yourself with a cosy blanket.

5. To come out of the pose, bend your knees towards your chest, roll over to your right side, press your hands onto the floor and walk yourself up to sitting, letting your head come up last.

6. Sit quietly for a few minutes before returning to your daily routine.

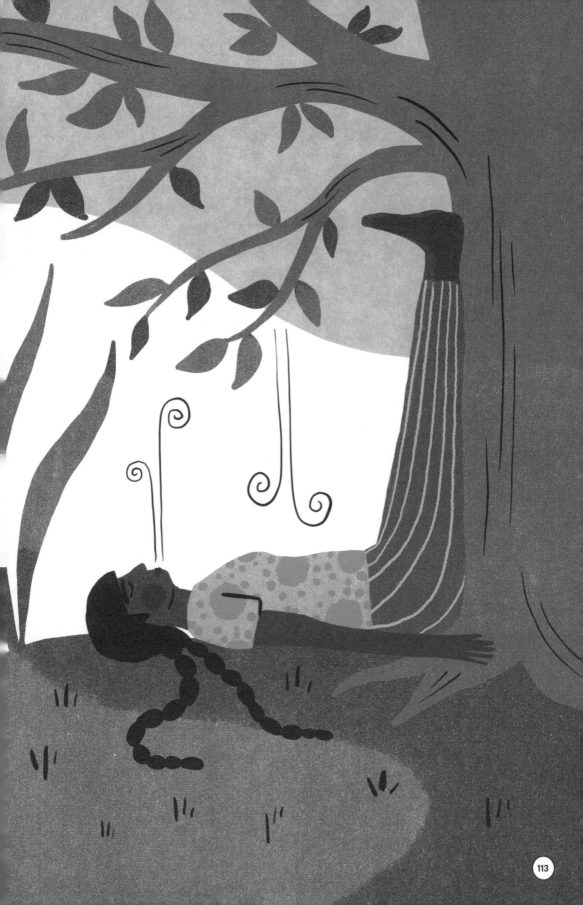

CORPSE POSE

Savasana

Despite its morbid name, Corpse pose firmly supports wellbeing and life. It releases tension and stress, lowers blood pressure, calms the mind and helps to bring balance to the nervous system. It's a great pose for finding stillness and calm through the limbs while surrendering to a peaceful moment.

Here's how to explore the pose:

1. From a seated position on your mat, lower your upper torso to lie flat.

2. Positioning your torso involves various stages. Start by relaxing and opening your hips outwards, tilting the pelvic region, which gently opens the legs. Feet extend away from each other. Legs are about hip-distance apart.

3. Gently lift and extend your shoulder blades backwards, opening your chest area. Allow your abdomen to release down into the mat.

4. Extend your arms gently outwards from the body, with palms open, fingers gently unfurling upwards.

5. Extend your neck and head away from your shoulders, tilt your chin towards your chest slightly to maintain a flat neck.

6. Soften and relax the muscles in your face, neck and tongue. Close or soften your eyes. You may choose to focus your gaze to the centre of your forehead.

7. When comfortable, bring your attention to your breath. Breathe in deeply and out slowly through your nose. Practise making the exhalation twice as long as the inhalation, for example, breathe in deeply for three counts, breathe out slowly for six.

8. As you consciously breathe, scan your body, beginning with your feet and working your way up to your head. With each out-breath, relax each muscle and body part.

9. Lie here and surrender to the peace within for between five and 10 minutes.

10. You may choose to listen to music or a guided meditation while in this state.

11. To come out of the pose, bring your attention back to your physical self, wiggle your fingers and toes and turn on your side to a foetal position. Rest for a few moments and then slowly come up to seated.

Tips:
* Wear clothes that will keep you warm but not overly hot.
* Place blankets or bolsters for added support where needed.

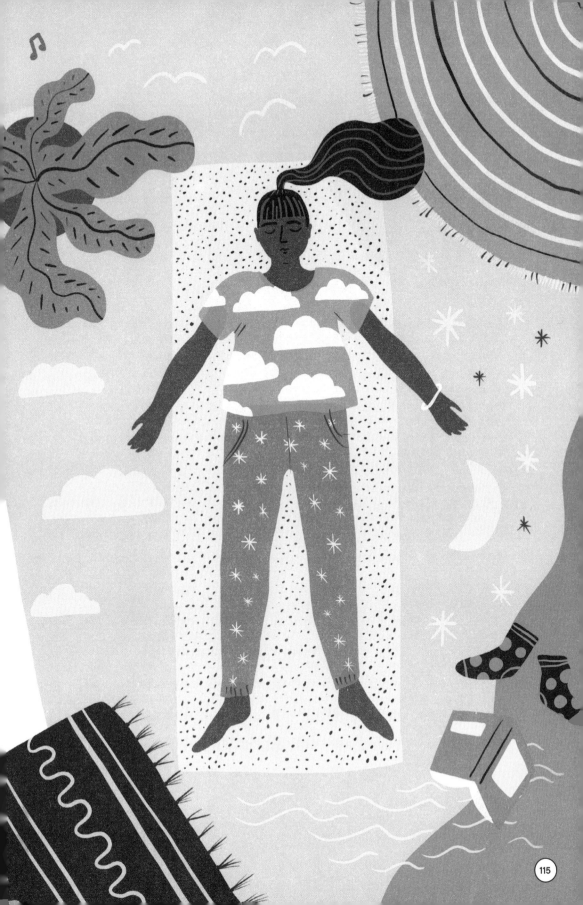

SUN SALUTATION

Surya namaskar

Known as the Sun salutation, this series of yoga poses is believed to date back 3,500 years to ancient India. It was traditionally a spiritual ritual used to honour the sun and was practised at either sunrise or sunset (or both). Sun salutation balances and energises the body, linking it with the breath and the mind, and revitalises the physical and spiritual self. It also strengthens and aligns the entire body, so it's a great way to prepare for a yoga session after you've performed a general warm-up (page 18). Have fun practising it in the morning before breakfast and observe how it energises you for your day.

Here's how to practise the sequence (continues overleaf):

1. Stand tall, holding your hands in Prayer pose (Step 6, page 21) at the heart centre. Take a few deep breaths and focus on the self, your core, your inner sun.

2. On an in-breath, circle your hands up above your head, reaching tall towards the sun. Look up to the sky through your open arms.

3. On an out-breath, flow your arms down in a circle around your body until the hands come to rest on the outside of each foot, with your fingers pointing forwards and aligned with your toes, as in Standing forward bend (page 24). You can bend your knees slightly, but keep the leg muscles engaged, as this will help to protect your back. Let your head hang gently towards the floor.

4. On an in-breath, bend your right leg and step back with your left, so you form a lunge position.

5. On an out-breath, step your right foot back to join the left, forming a straight line with your body in Plank (page 74).

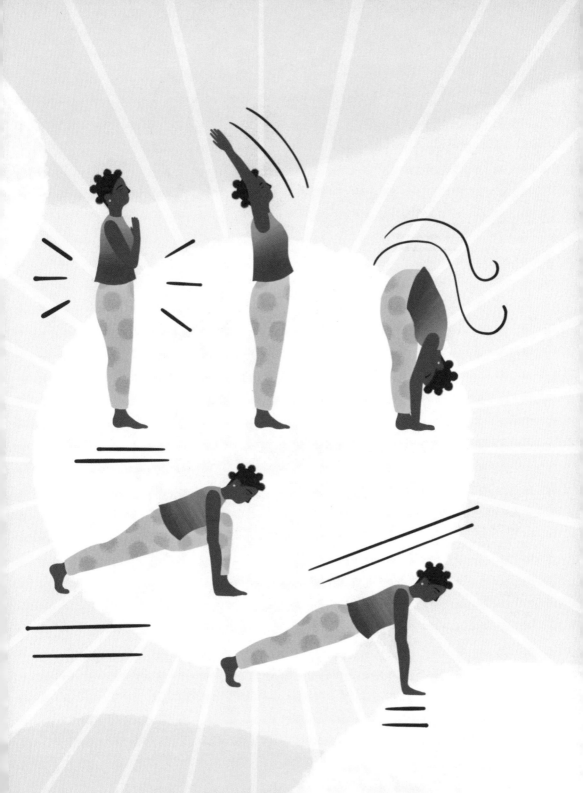

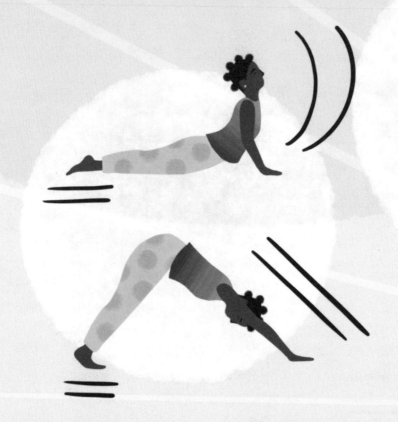

6. On an out-breath, lower your knees, chest and then chin to the floor. Keep your elbows tucked in near the body and palms flat on the floor, under the shoulders. On an in-breath, lift your chest upwards into Cobra (page 86), drawing your shoulders back. Take a few breaths here.

7. On an out-breath, tuck your toes under and push up into Downward-facing dog (page 72). Press down into the floor through your hands and feet while your hips pull upwards and backwards.

8. On an in-breath, step your left foot forwards between your hands, once again, forming a lunge position.

9. On an out-breath, bring your right foot forwards to join the left, coming back to Standing forward bend.

10. On an in-breath, circle your hands up round your body, and lift yourself to a tall standing position (your head comes up last). The hands join above the head in Prayer position.

11. On an out-breath, lower the hands to the heart centre and take a few deep, comfortable breaths.

12. When ready, repeat the sequence, this time leading with the right foot as you step back – and later forwards – into your lunge position.

13. You can repeat the sequence as many times as desired and at any time of day.

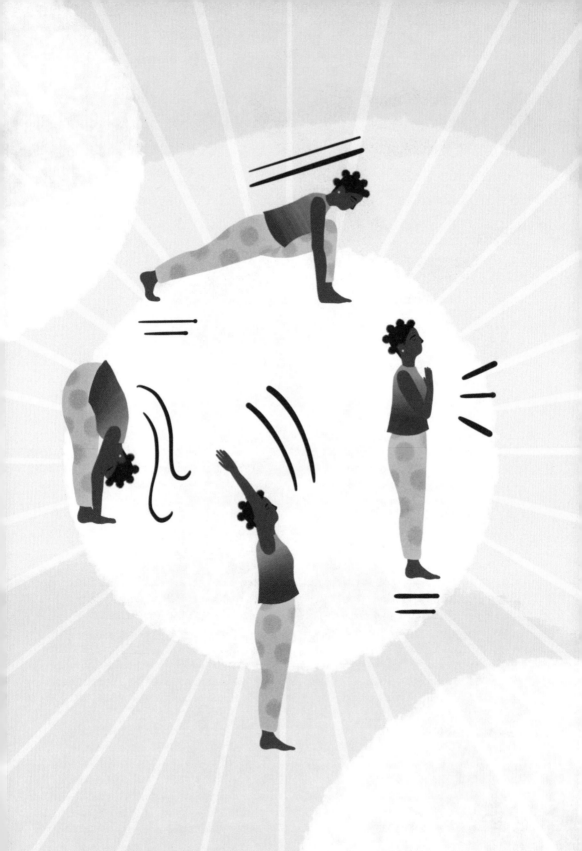

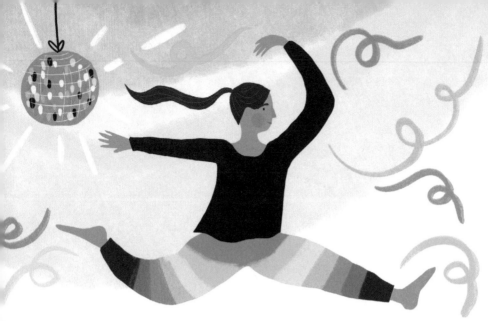

DANCE UP A STORM

If you'd like to introduce free expression into your practice, *Natya* yoga could be just your thing. Here's why, together with a fun sequence over the page

Sometimes it's good to shake things up a bit and there can be little doubt that *Natya* yoga does just that. A Sanskrit term, *Natya* means 'dance' and, when you combine it with *yoga*, which means 'union', you have a great pairing. Many indigenous cultures have used dance as a communion of the body, mind and spirit for centuries, so *Natya* yoga is similar in this respect.

In India, it has long been performed and taught by temple dancers and sages, confirming the spiritual connection between the two activities. Harnessing the art of dance and the practice of yoga can bring a host of physical, mental and spiritual benefits (see opposite).

Modern expression
When you break it down, dance is basically a sequence of movements performed in a rhythmic way, usually to music. Dance yoga, then, is a series of fluid yoga poses to the beat and tempo of song or sound, as you aim to reach a higher state of being.

There are many styles of dance and yoga, so it follows that there are many styles of *Natya* yoga to explore – something to suit all ages and interests. A broad taste in music can vary the mood and also give your practice a flexible range of rhythm, tempo, flow and energy.

Do try this at home
You could join one of the many classes, including hip-hop yoga, vinyasa dance, yoga trance dance and chair yoga dance. Or you may prefer to do your yoga rhythms at home, in which case there are many online videos you can follow. Just select your favourite songs or beats and get ready for dance yoga.

The lively, expressive movements raise more energy and heat within the body than other types of yoga, so keep a glass of water within reach. But other than that, it's your dance yoga practice, your choice of music, your means of expression. Get your groove on and enjoy the freedom.

Physical benefits

* Increases flexibility and helps to build muscle strength and tone.
* Improves respiration, energy and vitality, and cardio and circulatory health.
* Supports physical stamina.
* Releases stress and tension in the body, which can help boost the immune system.
* Promotes better posture and body awareness.

Mental benefits

* Boosts mood and self-esteem through the release of the feel-good hormone serotonin.
* Can help alleviate symptoms of anxiety and low mood.
* Activates sensory and motor circuits in the brain, which can help relieve stress.
* Improves spatial recognition and memory.

Spiritual benefits

* Symbolises the connection between the outer world and your own inner world.
* Can elevate emotions and energy flow to a higher state of consciousness.
* Provides space for your personal self-expression to flow.

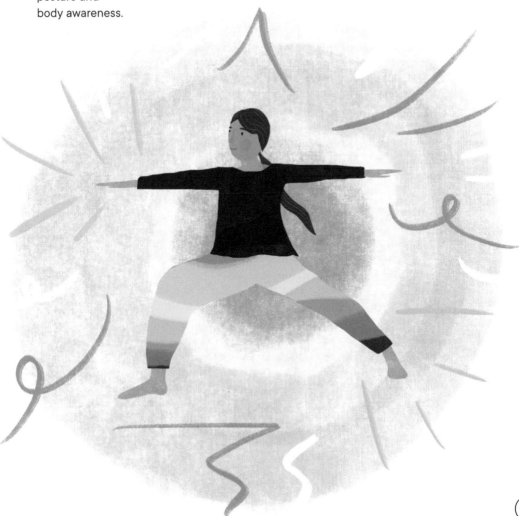

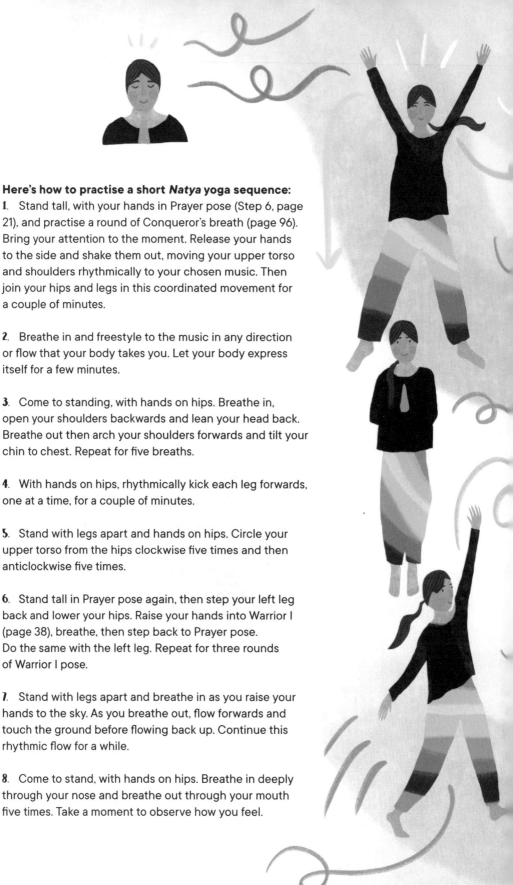

Here's how to practise a short *Natya* yoga sequence:

1. Stand tall, with your hands in Prayer pose (Step 6, page 21), and practise a round of Conqueror's breath (page 96). Bring your attention to the moment. Release your hands to the side and shake them out, moving your upper torso and shoulders rhythmically to your chosen music. Then join your hips and legs in this coordinated movement for a couple of minutes.

2. Breathe in and freestyle to the music in any direction or flow that your body takes you. Let your body express itself for a few minutes.

3. Come to standing, with hands on hips. Breathe in, open your shoulders backwards and lean your head back. Breathe out then arch your shoulders forwards and tilt your chin to chest. Repeat for five breaths.

4. With hands on hips, rhythmically kick each leg forwards, one at a time, for a couple of minutes.

5. Stand with legs apart and hands on hips. Circle your upper torso from the hips clockwise five times and then anticlockwise five times.

6. Stand tall in Prayer pose again, then step your left leg back and lower your hips. Raise your hands into Warrior I (page 38), breathe, then step back to Prayer pose. Do the same with the left leg. Repeat for three rounds of Warrior I pose.

7. Stand with legs apart and breathe in as you raise your hands to the sky. As you breathe out, flow forwards and touch the ground before flowing back up. Continue this rhythmic flow for a while.

8. Come to stand, with hands on hips. Breathe in deeply through your nose and breathe out through your mouth five times. Take a moment to observe how you feel.

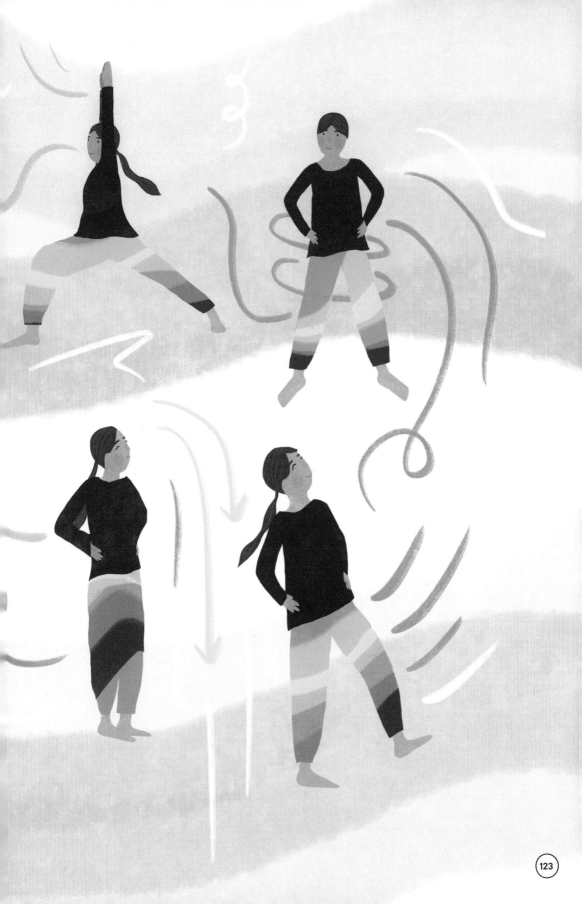

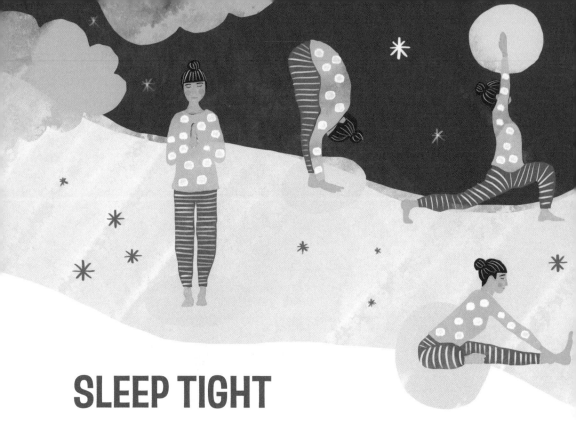

SLEEP TIGHT

A good night's rest is important for health and wellbeing – and sometimes yoga can ensure you get more of those valuable Zs. Here's a short flow movement to help you unwind from your day and prepare your mind and body for sleep

Here's how to practise the sequence:

1. Stand tall in Prayer pose (Step 6, page 21). Take between five and 10 Conqueror breaths (page 96), inhaling deeply through the nose and exhaling slowly out of your nose.

2. On an in-breath, raise your arms skywards. On an out-breath, fold into Standing forward bend (page 24). Bring your palms to rest on the ground next to your feet (bend your knees if that's more comfortable, but keep the back straight). Take a few breaths here.

3. On an in-breath, step your right leg back into a lunge, lift and roll back your shoulders and raise your hands skywards into Prayer pose, opening your chest forwards. Take a few breaths here. Step

back into Standing forward bend. Repeat, this time beginning with your left leg.

4. Come to sitting-up-tall position, legs stretched out in front of you. Breathing in, draw the right foot towards your pelvic region, placing its sole against the inside of your left thigh. Breathe out, then in, raising the arms skywards and folding forwards from the hips over your left leg, taking hold of your shin, ankle or left foot. Breathe here and release into the fold. On an in-breath, return to sitting tall, then release the right leg forwards. Repeat, this time on your other side.

5. Bending both legs in, draw your feet towards the pelvic region, then bring your soles together, knees opening away from

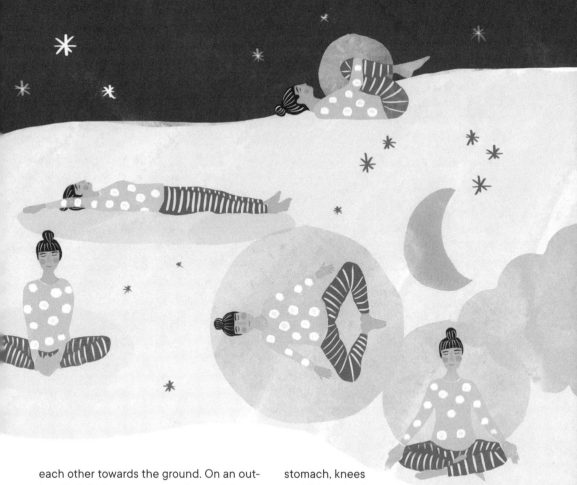

each other towards the ground. On an out-breath, fold the upper torso forwards from the hips. If you can, rest your head on the feet in Butterfly (page 46), but only fold as far as is comfortable. Take a few breaths.

6. Release the pose and lie down with your back flat on the ground. On an in-breath, stretch your arms along your ears away from the body and stretch your legs away from the body. Breathe here for a moment.

7. On an in-breath, bend your knees and draw them towards your torso to a position perpendicular – at an angle of 90 degrees – to your hips. Rest your hands on your knees or shins. On an out-breath, engage the muscles in the stomach and legs and draw your knees towards the chest. Keep your bottom, back, neck and head flat on the floor. On an out-breath, release the

stomach, knees and thighs back to perpendicular to the hips. Repeat this motion five times.

8. Return your legs to the outstretched position flat on the ground. On an in-breath, bend your knees and place your soles together, as close to the pelvic region as is comfortable. On an out-breath, release the knees and thighs to open away from each other, towards the ground in Reclining butterfly (page 68). Breathe here for a few moments.

9. When ready, release your legs back to an outstretched position, turn to the side and come up to seated. Place your hands in Prayer pose, a *mudra* – maybe touching thumb to forefinger on each hand – or rest them on your lap. Breathe and, if you wish, meditate here before going to bed.

INDEX

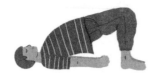

Page numbers for main descriptions are in bold.

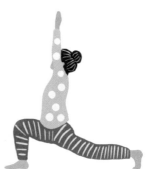

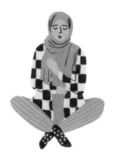

First published 2024 by
Guild of Master Craftsman Publications Ltd
Castle Place, 166 High Street, Lewes,
East Sussex BN7 1XU

ISBN 978 1 78145 486 2

Author and yoga advisor: Dawattie Basdeo
Guyana-born Dawattie is passionate about supporting and empowering young people
to manage their wellbeing. She has been teaching yoga for 14 years.

Editor: Catherine Kielthy
Designer: Jo Chapman
Editorial team: Josie Fletcher, Chloe Rhodes, Jane Roe, Yuliia Sytnikova
Publisher: Jonathan Grogan
Production: Jim Bulley

Illustrations: Sara Thielker

Colour origination by GMC Reprographics
Printed and bound in China

A Teen Breathe Publication

AMMONITE
PRESS

FSC
www.fsc.org
MIX
Paper | Supporting
responsible forestry
FSC® C016973

www.ammonitepress.com